# the total
# cancer
## wellness guide

# the total
# cancer
# wellness guide

## Reclaiming Your Life
## After Diagnosis

THE **WELLNESS** COMMUNITY

## Kim Thiboldeaux
*President and CEO*

AND

## Mitch Golant, Ph.D.
*Vice President, Research and Development*

BENBELLA BOOKS, INC.
DALLAS, TEXAS

BenBella Books, Inc.
6440 N. Central Expressway, Suite 617
Dallas, TX 75206
www.benbellabooks.com
Send feedback to feedback@benbellabooks.com

Printed in the United States of America
10 9 8 7 6 5 4 3 2 1

Library of Congress Cataloging-in-Publication Data

Thiboldeaux, Kim.
The total cancer wellness guide : reclaiming your life after diagnosis / by Kim Thiboldeaux, and Mitch Golant.
    p. cm.
    1. Cancer—Popular works. 2. Cancer—Psychological aspects. I. Golant, Mitch. II. Title.

    RC263.T45 2007
    616.99'4—dc22

                                                    2007006819

Proofreading by Emily Chauviere and Stacia Seaman
Cover design by Laura Watkins
Text design and composition by John Reinhardt Book Design
Index by Joanne Sprott
Printed by Bang Printing

Distributed by Independent Publishers Group
To order call (800) 888-4741
www.ipgbook.com

For special sales contact Yara Abuata at yara@benbellabooks.com

*This book is dedicated to the memory and vision of our dear friend and the founder of The Wellness Community, the late Dr. Harold Benjamin, and to all people affected by cancer.*

# Contents

# Acknowledgments

THE TOTAL CANCER WELLNESS GUIDE is a culmination of The Wellness Community's rich history. As we go to press, we celebrate twenty-five years of providing free services to cancer patients and their loved ones across the U.S. and around the globe. We are pleased to share our program philosophy, our lessons learned over the years, some helpful tips, and many enriching stories from our determined, passionate, funny, inspirational participants.

Many individuals have contributed to the writing of this book. To begin, we would like to acknowledge the tremendous wisdom and talents of our core team on the project: Patricia Ganz, M.D., Eunice Jadlocki, Katina Jones, and John Kleinbaum, Ph.D. In particular, Katina dedicated great energy, time, and passion to this project and brought extraordinary life experience and professional understanding to our work together. We would also like to thank our dear friends Dr. Mehmet Oz and Harriet Benjamin for their insights, which added greatly to the depth and clarity of the information. Your thoughtful perspectives have enhanced this guide for all people affected by cancer.

Next we would like to acknowledge the contributions of the entire TWC National Staff: Zena Itani, Vicki Kennedy, Janet McIver, Mark Meinke, Ellen Myerberg, Shannon Pao, Michelle Pollak, Lynn Ryker, Julie Taylor, Megan Taylor-Ford, and Erica Weiss. You are a top-notch team and it is an honor to work with you. Thank you also to all of our Wellness Community Executive Directors, Program Directors, Local Staff, Facilitators, Local and National Board Members, and Local and National Professional Advisory Board Members for your profound support of our mission and your unwavering support of this important project.

In addition, we would like to recognize the many corporations, foundations, and individuals who have provided critical financial support to The Wellness Community over the years. Your generosity has made our work possible.

We would also like to thank and acknowledge our friends and colleagues who made this project a reality: Ivan Kronenfeld, Carl Koerner, and Nathalie Casthely from Koerner and Kronenfeld Partners; Frank Weimann and his team at The Literary Group; Glenn Yeffeth and the team at BenBella Books; Andy Sandler, Ken Kaufman, and Matt Fagin at Skadden, Arps, Slate, Meagher & Flom, LLP; and, our dear friend and staunch supporter, Holly Page Hoscheit.

Finally, we would like to thank and acknowledge all those people affected by cancer who have attended our programs, both in person and online. You are the true inspiration for this book and you are the force that has led us to this work each and every day. We hope that The Wellness Community, in some small way, has touched you and helped you in your cancer journey.

—*Kim Thiboldeaux and Mitch Golant, Ph.D.*

WOULD LIKE TO THANK my many teachers, mentors, and guides along the way who have taught me always to seek purpose in my work and in my life and to dedicate myself wholly to any task I undertake, no matter how large or small. These include: Susan Cohen Smith, Warren Dennis (in memoriam), Ian Portnoy, Chris Wolf, Jeff Travers, Frank Condella, Kevin Rigby, Bill Ashbaugh, Harry and April Davidow, Jack Wickens, Chuck Scheper, Jill Durovsik, and Ellen Stovall.

I would also like to thank with all my heart my friends and family who have supported me in every phase of my life and have shown unparalleled excitement about this project. A special thank-you to my parents, Bert and Joann, for their love, their dedication to family, and the joy they exude each and every day.

Finally, I would like to thank my co-author on this project, Mitch Golant. Mitch has been at The Wellness Community practically since the beginning. His dedication and compassion are unmatched and his talents, beyond measure. Thank you, Mitch, for all that you do for people affected by cancer.

—*Kim Thiboldeaux*

I N April 1985, I began facilitating support groups at The Wellness Community. At that time, we were in a little yellow house in Santa Monica, California. None of us who were part of the licensed professional staff thought about our future. We were trying to understand The Wellness Community's Patient Active Concept. We were being taught by Harold Benjamin, Ph.D., TWC's founder. Today, Dr. Benjamin's seminal idea—the idea of the Patient Active—has permeated and positively influenced our understanding of how a patient's attitudes, actions, and beliefs impact the cancer experience. I had the great good fortune of having Dr. Benjamin as my mentor, friend, and partner for over twenty years. *The Total Cancer Wellness Guide* could not have been written without his teachings and dedication to all people with cancer.

I would also like to acknowledge my colleagues and friends throughout the psychosocial oncology field who have supported The Wellness Community's growth and progress over the last twenty-five years. In particular, I am grateful to David Spiegel, M.D., Janine Giese-Davis, Ph.D., Mort Lieberman, Ph.D., and Andy Winzelberg, Ph.D., who have mentored and taught me about doing research in a community setting. Kim and I are also deeply indebted to Deane Wolcott, M.D., Jimmie Holland, M.D., Matt Loscalzo, M.S.W., Julia Rowland, Ph.D., Barry Bultz, Ph.D., Alan Valentine, M.D., and Diana Jeffery, Ph.D., all of whom are masters in the science of caring. Thank you also to Joel DeGrands and Jeremy Lundberg for helping us serve cancer patients in a new and innovative way.

To my wife, Susan Golant, who has been my life partner and whose love and enduring support are at the heart of all things good and possible.

Lastly, my co-author Kim Thiboldeaux, whose tireless energy and belief that great good can come from our joining together in a common purpose is an inspiration and embodies true community.

—Mitch Golant, Ph.D.

# the total
# cancer
## wellness guide

THE NEWS ABOUT CANCER is better than ever. Even though more people are being diagnosed, fewer people are dying from the disease, and people are living longer and better with cancer. They're also learning how to live well with, through, and beyond it.

In the last twenty-five years, there have been dramatic advances in the diagnosis and treatment of cancer. These advances across most cancers have resulted in improved outcomes, leading to larger numbers than ever before of disease-free, long-term survivors, as well as prolonged survival for those who have developed *metastatic* diseases.

But as the number of those living with cancer rises, so does the burden on the healthcare system. As a result, patients are finding themselves in the position of having to take control of their own care plans. In essence, they have become empowered healthcare consumers. In a recent *New York Times*/CBS News poll of 1,111 adults in February 2005, 44 percent of patients who received a diagnosis sought more information about treatment options from sources who were not their physicians—including the Internet, friends, relatives, and even other doctors. Slightly more than half of surveyed patients who received a diagnosis were given multiple treatment options—and one-third made the decision on their own. Those between forty-five and sixty-four years old were most likely to take their medical care into their own hands by making informed, educated decisions about their treatments.

Patients need to work to overcome the three most common stressors from cancer: loss of hope, loss of control, and a sense of isolation. They must become educated and empowered. More than ever, today's cancer patient is captain of his or her own treatment team.

Still, unless cancer patients have effective support and resource teams in place to buffer against the trauma of the diagnosis and treatment, as well as to help navigate the many choices they have in every aspect of this life-transforming disease, they and their families will struggle daily with daunting decisions that most of us hope we will never have to

make. In many ways, it takes a village—a total cancer wellness community—to help guide the patient through the labyrinth of choices in dealing with issues ranging from dealing with the shock of initial diagnosis
to creating a living legacy and a meaningful life.

Through powerful, first-person testimonies from participants of The
Wellness Community worldwide, as well as a plethora of the best tips,
evidenced-based research, treatment, and support information currently available, *The Total Cancer Wellness Guide* will help you, the cancer
patient, feel empowered, positive, and focused on healing. You'll learn
how to live well with your disease—no matter what the road ahead may
bring.

Wherever you are in the continuum of the cancer experience (newly
diagnosed, in active treatment, in post-treatment, or a long-term survivor), this book has something to offer you. The Wellness Community's
Patient Active Concept is as relevant today as it was twenty-five years
ago—perhaps even more so.

—*Mehmet C. Oz, M.D.*, Chairman, Department of Surgery, New York
Presbyterian Medical Center; Director, Cardiovascular Institute, New
York Presbyterian Medical Center; and Professor of Surgery, Columbia
University

# The Wellness Community
## Twenty-Five Years and Growing

*The Wellness Community has been a precious part of my own cancer experience by helping me maintain a hopeful outlook on life. My group gave me the support and tools I needed to live well with cancer. I will always be thankful for The Wellness Community and their valuable online resources that helped me through my cancer experience.*

—ROSEANN FORZIANO,
*participant, The Virtual Wellness Community*

I N 1987, ROSEANN FORZIANO was a thirty-two-year-old wife and mother of an active four-year-old son. As a busy, young mom, the thought of having cancer was something that never entered her mind. However, after finding a lump in her right breast, she was diagnosed with breast cancer and had to face an uncertain future.

While searching for ways to cope with this unexpected and devastating turn of events, she read about Gilda Radner and her participation in The Wellness Community (TWC) of Santa Monica. Forziano also read Dr. Harold Benjamin's book, *From Victim to Victor*, and found The Wellness Community's honest and hopeful message for people with cancer critical to her own recovery.

Fifteen years later, in November 2002, Forziano's breast cancer returned. This time, she learned that she had stage IV breast cancer with metastases to the skin. She was terrified. Again, she turned to The Wellness Community, based in Washington, D.C., for inspiration and hope. Since she did not live close to one of the twenty-two TWC facilities around the country, she was fortunate to be able to rely on The Virtual

Wellness Community on the Internet for the information and support she needed.

Today, Forziano's cancer is under control, and she remains grateful to The Wellness Community and her online support group for giving her hope, inspiration, and a sense of well-being.

Like most of the more than 1.4 million cancer patients newly diagnosed each year—and the more than ten million cancer survivors—Forziano's life changed dramatically from the moment she was diagnosed. Suddenly, she was struggling to find her way through a swirling sea of paperwork, treatment options, and daunting decisions. The sad fact is, some doctors are too busy to offer personalized care, making the cancer experience seem even lonelier to patients like Roseann who feel their world crumbling around them.

## Enter The Wellness Community

Celebrating its twenty-fifth anniversary in June 2007, The Wellness Community is an international non-profit organization dedicated to providing free support, education, and hope to people with cancer and their loved ones. Through participation in professionally led support groups, educational workshops, nutrition and exercise programs, and mind/body classes, people affected by cancer learn vital skills that enable them to regain control, reduce isolation, and restore hope, regardless of the stage of their disease. Today, there are twenty-two Wellness Communities around the United States, twenty-eight satellite centers, two centers abroad in Tel Aviv, Israel, and Tokyo, Japan, five communities in development, and support online at The Virtual Wellness Community.

The Wellness Community was founded by Dr. Harold Benjamin in Santa Monica, California, in 1982. As a result of experience with his wife's breast cancer, and through subsequent years of study on the psychological and social impact of cancer, Dr. Benjamin formulated the Patient Active Concept. This revolutionary idea would be recognized years later at the Walt Disney World EPCOT Metropolitan Life exhibit as one of the most significant developments in the evolution of modern healthcare.

In addition to the Patient Active Concept, the other significant cornerstone of our program is that all services are provided free of charge in a home-like, community setting. "Community" is perhaps the most important aspect of The Wellness Community model of care that differentiates the program from any other. Today, thousands of people with cancer and their loved ones unite together through our programs. People come at diagnosis, during or at the end of treatment, at recurrence, or after several years out of treatment. They all come to learn that they are not alone in their fight—whether for physical, emotional, or spiritual recovery. Together, they regain a sense of control over their lives and ultimately discover that hope is a valuable tool irrespective of the stage of disease.

A significant factor in the expansion of facilities in the early 1990s can be directly attributed to Gilda Radner, a participant at TWC until her death from ovarian cancer in 1989. In her book, *It's Always Something*, she shares extensively about her experience at The Wellness Community. After reading her book, many patients have gone on to help bring a facility to their areas.

The national organization was officially formed in 1989 to facilitate expansion outside of California. In 2002, the national headquarters relocated to Washington, D.C., and The Wellness Community celebrated its twentieth anniversary. The national staff is leading The Wellness Community well into the future.

In order to accomplish our vision, The Wellness Community-National is committed to:

- Expanding public and professional awareness of The Wellness Community programs
- Strengthening existing facilities and developing new ones
- Providing state-of-the-art, evidence-based programs that are responsive to the needs of patients and families
- Participating in psychosocial research in order to evaluate our services and contribute to the greater professional body of knowledge about cancer and psychosocial support

In 2002, TWC launched The Virtual Wellness Community online at www.thewellnesscommunity.org. The Virtual Wellness Community delivers the first-of-its-kind, real-time online support groups led by trained professionals. The Virtual Wellness Community was developed as a result of TWC's groundbreaking pilot study with Stanford University and the University of California at San Francisco. This community-initiated research collaboration is the exact model about which the National Cancer Institute (NCI) is speaking for reaching underserved populations through evidenced-based research. TWC also serves teenagers with cancer in an award-winning Web-based program called "Group Loop" at www.grouploop.org.

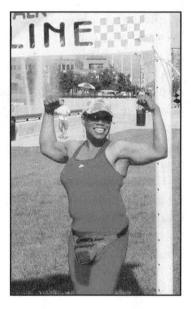

> *Every survivor or the loved one of a survivor I come into contact with, I give a pamphlet on TWC and a card. I let them know that TWC can really make a difference in how you go through your journey. I've visited TWCs around the country and the feeling is the same. I even do referrals to other TWCs around the country.*
>
> —Paula R. Davis,
> *participant,*
> *The Wellness Community -*
> *Central Indiana*

## About This Book

There are plenty of books available on the different forms of cancer. Some are clinical, while others are personal journeys from survivors offering advice on everything from choosing the right doctor to miracle cures. Like many other people with cancer, you might be looking for one book that tells you just about everything you need to know—in a positive, honest, and easy-to-understand manner. If so, you will most definitely benefit from the broad scope of detail The Wellness Community offers in this book. *The Total Cancer Wellness Guide* contains the facts about cancer, treatment options, and side effects management, without forgetting that you are a human being faced with major life issues hitting you with unimaginable voracity. More than anything else, you need to hear from others who have *really* been there, done that, and even lived to tell about it. Like them, you'll want to be an active participant in your own treatment—to grow from this experience and to regain your sense of control and hope.

## Guidance, Support, and Powerful Action Plans

If you or someone you love has recently been diagnosed with cancer, *The Total Cancer Wellness Guide* may be just what the patient ordered. This warm, accessible, and information-packed book is graced with the presence of dozens of The Wellness Community participants sharing their tips and personal observations about the entire cancer experience. It offers guidance and support every step of the way, empowering you to navigate your choices and make active decisions with the knowledge that it takes an entire community to achieve total wellness.

Broken into four sections that span the cancer management process from diagnosis through unpredictable future, *The Total Cancer Wellness Guide* is the first book to cover everything you and your family need to know about being active participants in your own long-term plan for well-being. With so many cancer patients becoming survivors, living longer and better has become an increasingly important point of focus for The Wellness Community and its team of experts.

At the end of each chapter, you'll find a Patient Action Plan with specific steps you can take now. These will help you put the main concepts expressed in each chapter to practical and immediate use.

With this new book, The Wellness Community aims to accurately and compassionately address all the physical, emotional, social, and practical needs of today's cancer patients, caregivers, and survivors—preparing you for wellness that can follow you throughout the rest of your life, regardless of how long that may be.

Join us at a Wellness Community near you—or anytime online at www.thewellnesscommunity.org. We're here for you!

> *[The Wellness Community's] wonderful group and facilitator helped me get through a very difficult time—emotionally and physically. So many available activities and resources to promote healing—and all without consideration of cost.*
>
> —LAWRENCE COHAN,
> *participant and survivor of stage III melanoma (currently in remission), The Wellness Community - West Los Angeles*

# Part One

# Becoming Patient Active

## Chapter 1

# What Is Cancer?

*Cancer changes many of the day-to-day aspects of living, but the pursuit of happiness can go on during the fight for recovery if you want it to.*

—HAROLD BENJAMIN,
*founder, The Wellness Community*

## A Brief History of Cancer

The National Cancer Act of 1971 declared a "War on Cancer" that started a significant crusade against a deadly disease. Since then, many strides have been made in improving early detection and developing safer and more effective treatments. Some cancers, such as Hodgkin's disease, specific leukemias, testicular, thyroid, and some childhood cancers, have had dramatic increases in cure rates. Yet, as our population ages, more and more people will continue to be diagnosed with cancer. This year, 1.4 million Americans will be diagnosed with cancer. In fact, one in two men and one in three women will be diagnosed in their lifetime. According to the National Cancer Institute, cancer has replaced heart disease as the leading cause of U.S. deaths for people under the age of eighty-five.

Increasingly, thanks to new discoveries in issues related to the psychosocial and physical challenges associated with cancer and its treatment, there is greater emphasis on quality of life, regardless of length of life. The Wellness Community has dedicated the last twenty-five years to addressing the issues of quality of life and the fight for recovery, in order to serve as an integral part of the medical care for people affected by cancer.

## Cancer Defined

Cancer occurs when:

- An abnormal cell appears in the body
- The cell continues to divide and subdivide after it should have stopped
- The new cells eventually form a clump, called a tumor. If unchecked, this clump will grow large enough to interfere with the delivery of nutrients and oxygen to nearby organs
- The abnormal, or cancer, cells are of the type that can survive in parts of the body other than where they originated

To explain in more detail, the human body is a collection of cells that perform separate, specific functions, each linked to the others, and operating in a highly regulated manner. In a normal cycle, a cell is born, matures, and performs its designated function, and then "dies." When a cell dies, it must be replaced by a new cell. This is accomplished when a nearby cell divides in two, and then those two divide, and so on, until the exact number of required new cells is achieved. Under normal circumstances, the birth and death of a cell is an exquisitely precise process.

Problems arise when, for reasons still unknown, a normal cell divides to replace other cells and gives birth to an abnormal cell. This abnormal cell does not stop dividing when it is supposed to and refuses to die on schedule. Such cells, if unchecked, divide and subdivide without end and eventually join together to form a tumor. As the tumor becomes larger, it impedes the functioning of nearby organs by intruding on their space and interfering with their supply of oxygen and nutrients. Eventually, unless the growth is stopped, or the tumor is removed, the healthy organs are destroyed.

There are two types of abnormal cells. The first can survive only at its place of origin and forms a tumor where it originates. This is called a *benign* tumor, which, while serious, can often be surgically removed, thereby ending the problem. The other type of abnormal cell, called a *malignant* tumor, is more dangerous because it cannot stop dividing when it is supposed to, and it can thrive any place in the body. This ability to travel and survive in other parts of the body is called *metastasis*. Cancer cells form a tumor at the primary site, as well as in places to which the tumor metastasizes.

Therefore, "cancer" is the generic name for more than 100 diseases that share similar characteristics of malignant cells. For cancer to be treated successfully, not only must the original tumor be controlled, but the spread of disease (metastasis) must also be stopped.

A leading contemporary theory states that abnormal cells may already be proliferating in our bodies as a normal course of our general health. The reason that these proliferating cells do not become cancerous may be that our immune systems are strong enough to destroy the cancer cells as they appear. Video has actually shown

> *This year, the U.S. government will spend about $14.4 billion in cancer research.*

cancer cells being attacked and destroyed by *immune system* cells, as if in battle. It's an inspiring sight. Some cancer patients use that image to visualize their bodies responding in a proactive manner.

## The Immune System: Our First Line of Defense

The immune system is an intricate system designed to protect the body from disease and from "foreigners" that invade through a break in the skin via food or other ingested matter, by way of the air we breathe, or through the rays to which we are exposed. For cancer to take hold, the cancer cell appears when the immune system is not strong enough to rid the body of that cancer cell. One way to think about cancer is that the cancer cell is not strong itself, but that the body's immune system is not strong enough to carry out its assigned job—removing cancer cells from the body. This view of cancer is generally known as the immune surveillance theory.

### Myths about Cancer
Despite the fact that cancer has been a leading cause of death for decades, not everything you hear about it is true. Take a closer look at the truths behind these popular misconceptions:

*Myth: Cancer is a death sentence.*
More than 60 percent of all people diagnosed with cancer today will be cured, and many others will continue to live with cancer as a manageable chronic condition

*Myth: You are powerless against cancer.*
There are actions, behaviors, and attitudes that you can use,

along with your physician and healthcare team, that will not only improve your quality of life but may enhance the possibility of recovery

*Myth: Surgery causes cancer to grow and spread.*
Surgery is often an important part of a successful treatment plan for cancer. Surgery and exposure to air do not affect the spread of cancer

*Myth: Disfiguring surgery is always part of cancer treatment.*
Some people with cancer need surgery, and some people do not. If you need surgery, you should know that reconstructive surgery techniques are used to avoid and correct disfiguring effects

*Myth: Terrible pain that cannot be relieved is part of cancer or its treatment.*
Some people do have pain with their cancer or treatment; other people do not. Most pain is treatable and can be relieved with modern pain relief medicine and other treatments

*Myth: Chemotherapy will make you sick each time you get it.*
There are many medications and other treatments that are now given to help control the side effects of chemotherapy. They help you feel and stay well during and after your chemotherapy treatment

*Myth: Radiation treatment burns off your skin.*
There are many skin care treatments and other medications that can be used for the beginning of your radiation. These treatments, used regularly, help manage the side effects of radiation

*Myth: Chemotherapy will always make your hair fall out.*
Only some chemotherapy makes you lose your hair, and even then, only temporarily. It grows back a few months after treatment and may look somewhat different than your hair did before treatment

*Myth: Having cancer and getting treatments means that you will be in the hospital all of the time.*
Most cancer treatment is given to you on an outpatient basis. Ask your doctor and nurse what you can expect from your treatment

*Before attending The Wellness Community, I saw cancer as a battle. TWC helped me to "embrace" my cancer. I know that sounds strange, but I no longer see my cancer as an ongoing battle, but [rather] something that's enhanced my life and helped me to appreciate every moment...something I wasn't doing before my cancer and my relationship with TWC. I used to say I wished there was an easier way to learn life's lessons...but now* I'm not so sure. No point in second-guessing....I just know life right now is incredible.

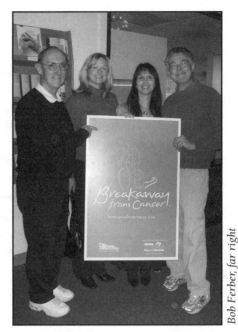

*Bob Ferber, far right*

—Bob Ferber,
*participant, The Wellness Community - Valley/Ventura*

## Gain Knowledge about Cancer Research Today

The National Cancer Institute has established a goal of minimizing the suffering and death due to cancer by 2015. Cancer research is rapidly changing, yet much work remains to be done. Andrew von Eschenbach, M.D., former director of the National Cancer Institute, states that it will be critical to "prevent the cancer process from occurring in the first place or detect the occurrence of cancer early enough to eliminate it."

In the meantime, new types and categories of drugs are being developed to treat the disease, and new mechanisms to better understand how the cancer cell functions at the most basic genetic level are being explored. While some cancers can be cured, others may never entirely disappear as a health problem and may require ongoing treatment to be controlled. As a result, patients are living longer, often with a better quality of life. In some types of cancer, it's becoming more of a chronic disease that must be managed and controlled over the course of many years and maintained until new discoveries in treatment are made. As a result of improved early detection and better cancer treatments, there are approximately 10.5 million cancer survivors alive today in the United States, compared to only 3 million people with a history of cancer who were alive in 1971.

For the last several decades, the common cancer treatment methods have been surgery, radiation, and chemotherapy. While these treatments are focused on destroying the tumor cells, they can damage normal cells in the process. The newest category of cancer treatments are *targeted therapies* that act in specialized ways to destroy or act against tumor cells, often not affecting normal cells. As a result, patients may experience less severe side effects. The newer treatments can also be combined with older therapies to enhance anti-tumor effectiveness. Details about targeted therapies, including those impacting cell growth and death, hormones, the immune system, and aspects of genes, can be found later in this book.

**Patient Action Plan**
- Gain as much knowledge as you can as soon as you discover you have cancer
- Learn from others who have been there by joining a support group as early in the process as possible
- Know that knowledge is power in the fight against cancer
- Understand that cancer research is an ongoing process, and new treatments are always on the horizon
- Learn to become more comfortable with the idea of asking your doctor more questions

## Chapter 2

# Diagnosis and Beyond

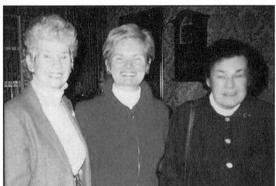

*Eileen O'Donnell, center*

*One sleet gray March day, the color of dying ashes, the sky the color of Mark Twain's mustache, [my doctor] announced: 'You have cancer.' My face turned gray.... I heard distinctly, 'You are going to die.'*

—EILEEN O'DONNELL, *self-described "cancer-thriver" and participant,* The Wellness Community - Greater Lehigh Valley

■ F YOU'VE JUST BEEN diagnosed with cancer, chances are you're in a state ▌ of shock. Often, the mere mention of the word "cancer" causes alarm. ■ At the very least, it causes us to stop in our tracks as we struggle to come to terms with the impact this diagnosis will have on our lives.

Sometimes, depending on how much we know about cancer in general, or through experience that we may have from dealing with cancer in others, we may consider a cancer diagnosis tantamount to a death sentence. We may panic, assuming that the only news is going to be bad news. This reaction is natural, but it's not likely to be the truth of the situation in today's world, when more and more cancers are being treated more successfully.

What can you do if you've just been diagnosed? First, take a deep breath. Realize that you're the same person you were just a moment ago, before cancer entered your consciousness. Second (and this isn't meant to seem contradictory), realize that the one thing you *can* expect is that cancer will change your life. Some things may actually be better than before; cancer can bring certain gifts to us. Conversely, your circumstances may change in ways you consider less positive. Either way, the sooner you can adjust to the fact that your life has changed, the sooner you can participate more fully in managing your illness.

It's natural to expect your first reactions to be shock, grief, panic, and resistance to the changes occurring in your life. But the good news is that there are practical steps you can take that will help you regain a sense of control over your circumstances. There are ways to regain your emotional balance. You can *still* be the person in the driver's seat of your life. You can control your response to the illness. You can find positives along the way, throughout your journey with this disease called cancer.

And what a journey it will be! One minute you were living your life, seemingly on your own terms. In an instant, all of that changed. It's as if your life was swept up into a tornado, leaving you standing amid the pieces of your old self, now in total disarray.

But you're not alone on this journey. You're actually the nucleus of a brand-new team—a team devoted to taking the best possible care of you. True, you didn't choose this journey, but it will nevertheless be brightened by the love and concern of your family and friends, plus new friends you'll meet along the way, including other patients and a host of medical professionals who may become part of an "unofficial" extended family.

## What a Cancer Diagnosis Means...and Doesn't Mean

In the last twenty-five years, there have been dramatic advances in the diagnosis and treatment of cancer. Advances across most cancers have resulted in improved outcomes, leading to larger numbers of disease-free, long-term survivors, as well as prolonged survival for those developing metastatic diseases. Nearly 1.4 million cancer survivors living today were diagnosed more than twenty years ago—and that's not a misprint.

This dramatic progress was brought about by ongoing new discoveries in the diagnosis and treatment of cancer. Additionally, those diagnosed today benefit from the medical profession's increased awareness and understanding of the psychological impact that a cancer diagnosis and treatment have for the patient and his or her loved ones.

Despite great improvement in the early detection and treatment of many cancers, a diagnosis of cancer can instill fear and anxiety in the person getting this news. It's true that cancer can disrupt daily life, including family, work, education, friendships, and finances. Research has shown that, in general, 25–30 percent of newly diagnosed and recurrent patients experience elevated levels of emotional distress. Some individuals may require psychiatric intervention to help them deal with the diagnosis.

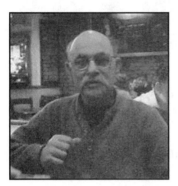

*I have heard cancer survivors say they have been blessed. I totally agree and have found new meaning to life, to relationships, and to giving. All material things are just that— things—but relationships are forever. I have permanently gone from handshakes to hugs for my friends and family.*

—Joe Hendrix,
*participant, The Wellness Community -
South Bay Cities*

## Acknowledge the Change Cancer Has Brought to Your Life

Can anything be done to counteract such distress? In a word, yes. In fact, you'll find a long list of coping skills at your disposal. One key to dealing with this change in your life is to acknowledge it. Rant and rave if you need to. Cry. Laugh. Verbally express your anger, dismay, fear, and other emotions. But find some way to acknowledge that your life has changed…and that you wish it wouldn't. That one action will help to dispel some of the stress you're feeling.

Some people with cancer actually create an irreverent nickname for the illness, or they refer to events in their life as "BC" (before cancer) or "AC" (after cancer). They do this to incorporate the illness as part of their lives—because it's just "part of" their lives. The secret to a healthy mindset is contained in those two little words: "part of."

Failing to acknowledge the changes in your life post-cancer can allow the illness to loom so largely that it seems insurmountable. Acknowledging its presence doesn't mean you're granting it permission to take over your life. Stay in the driver's seat by saying, in effect, "I see you. I'll deal with you, but you don't get to become my entire life. I'm still going to be the boss."

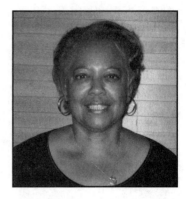

*I joined The Wellness Community after my first surgery at City of Hope. I became aware of the devastating effects cancer has on so many others. As we shared stories and experiences, I learned so much about the healthcare system, doctors, nurses, and hospitals. I not only became better informed, I also learned how to ask the right questions. I was also able to find a Web site with other people who had my same kind of cancer. Between the TWC support group and my online group, I became educated in cancer lingo and actively sought the care I needed.*

—DIANE TURNER,
*participant, The Wellness Community - Foothills*

## Become Informed

One of the most important tools for reducing emotional stress and being a proactive partner in your own care is information. You and your family need reliable, comprehensive, and current information to help identify the best options for treatment, to manage the disease better over time, and to feel confident that you're receiving the best possible care available.

A person diagnosed with cancer today is supported by help, hope, and information. Knowledge, it is said, is power. Educate yourself or, if that's too difficult, designate a friend or family member to gather information and distill it for you.

*It's not a sign of weakness to say to yourself and others that you have cancer, that you wish you didn't, and that it's simply an ongoing "part of" your life.*

A generation ago, cancer was often a dark secret that we kept to ourselves and our closest family members; indeed, some people diagnosed in bygone times often didn't tell their families about it, and some family members kept the truth from their loved one who had the disease.

Today's patients are fortunate to have access to much more information about their disease and its treatment than patients did one or two generations ago. Obtaining and assessing that wealth of information is very important. Those living with cancer have the opportunity to be savvy consumers, starting with becoming knowledgeable about their own situation. You're encouraged to form a partnership with your medical team, versus simply being a passive "body" receiving treatment.

The amount of information available to you can frankly be overwhelming, both in its content and complexity. That's why it's important to have a team of helpers working with you. Is one family member easily able to negotiate the maze of insurance forms on your behalf? If so, let the relative do so. Is a good friend a calming influence on you when you're visiting your doctor? Ask that friend to accompany you and to act as your "scribe." He or she can take notes while you talk with and listen to your physician.

Often, an outsider such as a trusted friend is much better at gathering vital information at such times—and much less prone to the up and down emotions you and your closest family members may be experiencing. Having someone take notes at appointments leaves you free to concentrate fully on what's being said. You don't need to worry about getting it wrong or about not remembering the details of the conversation. Having someone accompany you to appointments means you have a team member who, when all you can remember are fears or worries, can say, "Don't you remember? The doctor said you're very unlikely to develop that symptom."

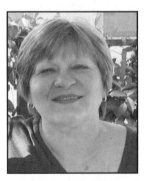

*I was a very healthy person until I was diagnosed with cancer. I never had any symptoms, so when I went to the doctor because I started bleeding, I told him I supposed I had hemorrhoids. The same day I was told by my doctor I had cancer. My family and I were very worried about my future. The days were very long until my surgery. My surgeon was excellent, the surgery was successful, and [the surgeon] was so optimistic that he promised me I would see my grandchildren, which made me much more relaxed.*

—KATHARINA PEREZ,
*participant, The Wellness Community -
San Francisco East Bay*

## Get Organized

Of course, the sheer volume of information available about your illness can be perplexing. Sometimes it's rather technical, even when it's supposed to be user-friendly. Sometimes one source will contradict another, and you may wonder which one is "right" or more reliable. You'll also find that the information base grows exponentially. Every time you think you understand the basics of your disease, a new treatment or a new article comes to light and takes you down another tangent. Or someone innocently and unknowingly shares information that's inaccurate. It can all be quite bewildering.

That's why, in addition to having someone take notes at appointments, it's helpful to have someone keep track of all of the information. After all, the information can't be very effective if it's simply lying in piles all around the house; some system of organization is needed.

Perhaps someone can file the information you receive. Separate sections might include "Practical Information" (example: directions to the treatment center or the appropriate parking deck); "Side Effects," if you're undergoing new treatment; "Prescriptions," which could be a list of medications you're taking; and so on.

You might also ask your spouse or a friend to take charge of other aspects of your new "living-with-cancer" world. For example, someone could become the "go-to" person to provide updates to friends and associates about your condition, at least at times when you're too busy or too tired to deal with these conversations. This same person could help you set up an online group of your own in which to communicate with family and friends who are far away—or they could simply e-mail you the latest research on treatment options.

Choose someone you know you can depend on to help organize childcare, meals, laundry, and other aspects of everyday life, at least in times when you may not be feeling well enough to do so yourself. If you're open to such assistance, you need only ask for it, because many friends and relatives will likely ask for ways they can help, anyway. If you don't have such resources among your friends and family, often someone on your medical team, such as a medical social worker, can refer you to groups that provide hands-on help to cancer patients.

## Partner with Your Healthcare Team

Throughout this book, reference is often made to the importance of forming an effective partnership with your healthcare team. Being able to communicate effectively with your medical team will yield dividends in the form of optimal treatment and the building of trust and confidence in your medical professionals. It's the best way to ensure your emotional and physical wellness throughout your treatment process.

## Fight Hopelessness

Sometimes, the type and severity of the cancer and/or its treatment can create feelings of despair for the individual with cancer, as well as for his or her loved ones. For example, a study published in 2001 reported that people with lung cancer, as a group, experienced the highest levels of emotional distress, followed by people with brain tumors or pancreatic cancer. This study and others demonstrate the need for support services for people with cancer and underscores the need for psychosocial screening to determine the level of distress and the risk of emotional difficulties for people with cancer.

Just as scientists are working to discover how to detect cancer earlier, psychosocial oncology professionals would like to help identify emotional distress or other social and emotional concerns early on in your diagnosis so that you can get the support you need to participate actively in treatment and maintain a good quality of life throughout cancer and beyond.

Feeling distress, or even hopelessness, can have many different dimensions. It's not easily described as one single emotional or physical reaction. Distress, as it relates to a person with cancer, focuses on describing or measuring the unpleasant emotional experiences that can impact cognitive, behavioral, social, emotional, and spiritual functioning, and may also interfere with the person's ability to cope effectively with cancer, its physical symptoms, and its treatment.

Distress can range from very common feelings of vulnerability, sadness, or fear to problems that can become more disabling, such as depression, anxiety, panic, social isolation, and existential or spiritual crisis.

The good news is that feelings and concerns are entirely manageable with proper support and screening. Distress can be assessed and managed according to clinical practice guidelines. A key ingredient to appropriate management, of course, is for you to be candid in describing your feelings to your medical team.

## Don't Blame Yourself

It would seem obvious that you aren't to blame for your illness, but in our society today, too many individuals want to place blame and many people, sadly, blame themselves for things that are truly beyond their control. Cancer is a good case in point.

Your lifestyle or some of the choices you've made can certainly impact your immune system negatively, but how can you be sure that's really what happened? Perhaps your immune system may be more susceptible to cancer cells than someone else's. You might have a genetic predisposition to a certain disease, and it's possible that no prevention tactic or positive lifestyle choices would have made a difference.

Unless you were given a 100 percent chance of developing cancer and chose not to make changes to avoid it, you can't be held responsible for having cancer. And of course, even if you *did* know that you were opening yourself to an increased risk of cancer, you can't be sure that any different behavior on your part would have guaranteed a different outcome.

This is important because the last thing you need in addition to your cancer is an unfair burden of guilt. Blaming yourself can actually be more hazardous to your health. Dr. Harold Benjamin, founder of The Wellness Community, notes: "If you blame yourself, you may trigger two other self-defeating reactions: You may unconsciously forgo taking actions in your fight for recovery, and you may inhibit the spontaneous self-healing responses your body would automatically take to return to its normal condition."

So, give yourself a break. Deal with today's realities, not yesterday's regrets. Today is all any one of us has, truly.

> *You do not realize it immediately, but once you're diagnosed with cancer, you are changed. From that moment forward, you'll always be one of two things: either a cancer patient or a cancer survivor. But in either case, 'cancer' is one-half of your title. I am not pleased I got cancer; however, as a result of the challenge, I'm more focused and cognizant of everything in my life that is of value.*
>
> —Drew Van Dopp,
> *participant, The Wellness Community - Delmarva*

## Use Laughter as Medicine

Most of us are familiar with the old saying: "Laughter is the best medicine." One reason such axioms have become popular and continue to be used is that they contain some truth. That's definitely the case about laughter being healthy for us.

More and more research is being done about the health benefits of laughter. A good laugh releases healthy endorphins that help to lighten depression, reduce discomfort, and help in the healing process. More than twenty-five years ago, before most experts understood the value of laughter in healing, Norman Cousins—a writer, author, and the long-time editor of *Saturday Review*—dealt with his own life-threatening illness by using laughter as a healing tool. He maintained a positive attitude and daily watched comedies—often, the Marx Brothers—on television and on tape. He laughed often and made sure to enjoy a hearty belly laugh several times each day.

All that laughter had its effect. Cousins's bestselling book, *Anatomy of an Illness as Perceived by the Patient*, reveals that the author's illness—plus a heart condition developed later—was kept at bay, perhaps even cured, by his regimen of positive emotions and laughter. Of course, there may have been other factors in his seemingly miraculous recovery, but Cousins's story is only one of many hailing the health benefits of laughter.

## Gilda's Legacy of Love and Laughter

*I stopped sitting at home saying, 'Why me?' I began to crawl to The Wellness Community like someone in search of an oasis in the desert. My car couldn't get there fast enough to be nourished by other cancer patients and to know that I was not alone.*

—GILDA RADNER,
*It's Always Something*

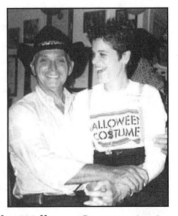

Comedienne Gilda Radner, who came to The Wellness Community in Santa Monica when she was diagnosed with ovarian cancer, took a similar approach. Terminally ill, she still found much about which to laugh in life. She even wrote a book, *It's Always Something*, a frank description of living with cancer, told in her inimitable humorous style. Radner's determination to continue being funny and to live fully and as long as possible has been an inspiration for thousands of people who are living with cancer.

"When Gilda was first diagnosed, she withdrew from everyone," said Pam Zakheim, who grew up with Radner and founded The Wellness Community-Boston at the late comedienne's request. "The difference between the day before she went to The Wellness Community and the day after her first visit was like night and day. Her hope was revitalized, as was her sense of self. She started communicating with her friends and family again. It was really quite inspiring."

Throughout the rest of her illness, Radner always remembered the lessons she had learned at The Wellness Community. "There will always be blood tests and X-rays and CAT scans and uncertainty," she said in her 1988 book. "The goal is to live a full, productive life, even with all that ambiguity. No matter what happens, whether the cancer never flares up again, or whether you die, the important thing is that the days that you have had, you will have *LIVED*. It's a hard concept, and it doesn't mean denying the depression and anger that come with cancer. But I've learned what I can control is whether I am going to live a day in fear and depression and panic, or whether I am going to attack the day and make it as good a day, as wonderful a day, as I can."

### Join a Club . . . Just for Laughs

A relatively new concept, laughing clubs, was created in 1995 by Dr. Maden Kataria and his wife, Madhuri, of India. Today, these clubs are found worldwide—at healthcare centers, workplaces, assisted living facilities, schools, senior centers, and health clubs—basically, anywhere people want more laughter. Groups meet weekly in some areas, and the only item on the agenda is to laugh.

So, it seems that guffaws and giggles are healthy in themselves for all of us, but they also serve as a way to keep cancer in its place. If it can't keep us from laughing and being ourselves in as many ways as possible, then we're not victims. After a cancer diagnosis, it's important to keep reminding yourself that you can still be *YOU*. Laughter is one of the tools

that can help relieve stress—but it can also help you stay emotionally healthy throughout and beyond your treatment.
For more information, visit www.laughteryoga.org.

**Patient Action Plan**
- Acknowledge the change that cancer has brought to your life
- Become informed
- Get organized
- Partner with your healthcare team
- Fight hopelessness
- Don't blame yourself
- Use laughter as medicine

*Chapter 3*

# Patient Active
## The Wellness Community Approach

*People with cancer who participate in their fight for recovery, along with their healthcare team, rather than acting as hopeless, helpless, passive victims of the illness, will improve the quality of their lives and may enhance the possibility of recovery. The Patient Active Concept combines the will of the patient with the skill of the physician—a powerful combination in the fight against the common enemy, cancer.*

—THE WELLNESS COMMUNITY'S PATIENT ACTIVE CONCEPT

N 1982, THE WELLNESS COMMUNITY was founded by Dr. Harold Benjamin based upon the *Patient Active Concept*: adopting a set of actions, behaviors, and attitudes that will improve the quality of a cancer patient's life and could, therefore, enhance the possibility of recovery.

Mostly, being *Patient Active* is about feeling and acting empowered. It's about *active participation* in the choices you make with your healthcare team. It's about being *actively aware* of the medical standard of care, new discoveries in cancer, and ways to manage side effects. It's about active involvement in all aspects of your cancer experience.

Choosing to be Patient Active is not about one monumental decision, but rather a series of small, incremental choices. These choices help you regain a sense of control over your treatment and your life in general.

There's no right or wrong way to be Patient Active, because in this model, you decide what's best for you. You make informed decisions about your own treatment, the management of your side effects, and the

31

issues pertaining to your emotional well-being. This includes strengthening your relationships with others as well as coping with the stress that cancer brings into your life.

Being Patient Active means you're empowered to take specific steps to help reduce feelings of *unwanted aloneness*, *loss of control*, and *loss of hope*. This book includes information to address some of those stressors by learning more about the newest advances in cancer treatment and emotional support—including support groups and other programs at The Wellness Community nearest you, or online at: www.thewellnesscommunity.org.

## Form a Partnership with Your Physician

Because a good relationship with the right physician is a critical part of your Patient Active plan, you need to focus some time and energy into achieving such a relationship. Here are some steps to get you on the road to a productive, Patient Active partnership:

- **Step One: Choose a medically competent physician.**
  In most cases, this is done by recommendation and reputation. There are also situations in which your insurance carrier or health maintenance organization (HMO) will select your physician
- **Step Two: Ensure that the relationship is, at the very least, cordial.**
  It does not have to blossom into a full-blown friendship for it to be effective and efficient. It's only necessary that it be agreeable
- **Step Three: Make sure that the expectations of both you and your doctor are clearly understood by each of you.**
  Some patients want every bit of information and detail they can get, while others prefer to stick to the high points. Make sure that your doctor knows how much you want to know—and how much involvement you really want or need to have in your treatment plan
- **Step Four: If your needs as a patient conflict seriously with the doctor's, consider whether it's in your best interest to find another physician.**
  Many people find it embarrassing or difficult to leave a physician. Yes, it can be a drastic step, but it's not unthinkable, nor should it be impossible. If you feel you're at an impasse, it's likely that this is the most appropriate step. Often, cancer patients are

treated by a group of physicians that may include an *oncologist*, *radiologist*, surgeon, and/or another kind of specialist, along with the family doctor. A frequent complaint is that no one seems to be in charge—each physician acts almost independently, and there's no one from whom the patient can get all of the information they need to make a decision. To be Patient Active, you must encourage one of the doctors to serve as coordinator of the team and keeper of all information. This should be your point person throughout treatment

> *I had a decision to make about which treatment course to take. I conducted my own survey on how well myeloma patients were doing after stem cell transplants. The answer was not very well, as far as I was concerned. In many cases after the transplant, the cancer returned within twelve to eighteen months. The oncologists recommending stem cell transplants were telling patients that this procedure would give them 'more time,' but my conclusion doubted this...and with what quality of life? I decided not to have a stem cell transplant. My condition has been stable for three and a half years, and my blood numbers are almost normal. In spite of having cancer and dealing with chronic pain, I've managed to travel to Italy, Alaska, California, Florida Keys, Arizona, Mexico, and the Caribbean four times. I actually celebrated my seventieth birthday, which I thought I would never see, in Las Vegas last year.*

> —J. DONALD DETENBER,
> *participant, The Wellness Community - Greater Boston*

**The Wellness Community Patient/Oncologist Statement**
As your physician, I will make every effort to:
- Provide you with the care most likely to be beneficial to you
- Inform and educate you about your situation, and the various treatment alternatives. How detailed an explanation is given will be dependent upon your specific desires
- Encourage you to ask questions about your illness and its treatment, and answer your questions as clearly as possible. I will also attempt to answer the questions asked by your family. However, my primary responsibility is to you, and I will discuss your medical situation only with those people authorized by you

- Remain aware that all major decisions about the course of your care will be made by you. However, I will accept the responsibility for making certain decisions if you want me to
- Assist you in obtaining other professional opinions if you desire, or if I believe it to be in your best interest
- Relate to you as one competent adult to another, always attempting to consider your emotional, social, and psychological needs, as well as your physical needs
- Spend a reasonable amount of time with you on each return visit, unless required by something urgent to do otherwise, and give you my undivided attention during that time
- Honor all appointment times unless an emergency arises
- Return phone calls as promptly as possible, especially those you indicate as urgent
- Make test results available promptly if you desire such reports
- Provide you with any information you request concerning my training, experience, philosophy, and fees
- Respect your desire to try treatment that might not be conventionally accepted. However, I will give you my honest opinion about such unconventional treatments
- Maintain my active support and attention throughout the course of the illness

As the patient, I will:
- Comply with the agreed-upon treatment plan
- Be as candid as possible about what I need and expect from my medical team
- Be honest about wanting or needing another professional opinion, as well as other forms of therapy in which I am involved
- Honor all appointment times unless an emergency arises
- Be as considerate as possible when it comes to my doctor's need to be with other patients
- Make all phone calls to my doctor during working hours. I will call at night or on weekends only when absolutely necessary
- Coordinate the requests of my family and friends, so that all questions can be answered by my doctor at one time

*—adapted from a draft by oncologists Richard Steckel, Michael Van Scoy Mosher, Laurence Heifetz, and Fred P. Rosenfelt*

*I didn't realize how precious life can be until the day my wife informed me that she had been diagnosed with stage III breast cancer. I had a very difficult time believing that she could have developed cancer. However, we both accepted it, and after consulting with our medical team, we felt we could defeat the cancer if we could establish a positive attitude during the treatment phase of the disease. We found the Pasadena Foothills [TWC] staff to be an excellent source of information... without the help of TWC, life would have been more difficult, and progress toward recovery more painful. Thank you very much!*

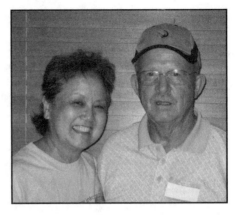

—CHARLES HOLLOWELL,
*caregiver participant, The Wellness Community - Foothills*

## Regain a Sense of Hope and Control

According to Harold Benjamin, Ph.D., The Wellness Community's founder, hope consists of three elements: a desire that an event will take place, the possibility that the event will occur, and the belief that you will be pleased if it does. Hopelessness, he said, consists of only two elements: desire that an event will take place and the belief that, no matter what you do, there is no possibility that the event will occur. "As you can see, hopelessness always includes a feeling of helplessness. In most cases of cancer, neither hopelessness nor helplessness is realistic, although the myths of cancer would fool you into thinking otherwise," Dr. Benjamin said. "As a matter of fact, in the great majority of cases, it's unreasonable and unrealistic *not* to have hope."

### Are You Feeling Hopeless?
If you're not sure, ask someone close to you to answer the following questions:

- Have I been using negative words that indicate a feeling of doom?
- Have I been acting as if there's no reason for hope?
- Do I appear to be moving away from the people I love—and those who love or care about me?
- Treatment notwithstanding, do I seem more listless and lethargic than usual?

Lack of hope can be a serious matter for the cancer patient. Studies show that loss of hope is one of the most debilitating psychological problems cancer patients face, along with unwanted aloneness and loss of control. But how do you maintain your sense of hope and control after a cancer diagnosis?

First of all, it's important to remember that there are more people than ever before who are considered completely recovered, meaning there's no evidence of the illness, and they have the same life expectancy as someone who has never had cancer. The fact is, every cancer has a recovery rate—so the outcome of your particular type of cancer isn't certain.

Other ways to regain a sense of hope include: using stress-management techniques (*see Chapter 7*), connecting with others whose lives have been impacted by cancer (*see Chapter 14*), keeping up with your regular social contacts and interactions, using hopeful and optimistic words about your illness, and, most importantly, making plans for the future. There's no reason *not* to do so!

Although no one can promise complete recovery, hope is there for the taking—and with hope comes an improved quality of life, which, as Dr. Benjamin said, "is a reasonable goal in itself."

**Patient Action Plan**

The following guidelines are designed to help you more thoroughly understand the instructions given to you at each visit with your doctor, as well as increase your peace of mind while building trust and confidence in your doctor:

- Before the visit, prepare a written list of the questions you want to ask your doctor. This will ensure that your questions get asked—and answered
- For the same reasons, prior to your visit, prepare a written list of the information you want your doctor to know
- If you don't understand something your doctor says, say

so. If you don't speak up, you may wind up following the wrong advice or taking an improper dosage of medication

- Take someone with you when you go to the doctor. Your friend or family member will not be as stressed as you and will be able to listen and understand the doctor with greater objectivity
- Get a second opinion when a major course of action is contemplated
- Decide with your physician who is to make the final decision as to treatment, or if you will make that decision together

Most important, comply with the instructions of your physician. It's estimated that only 50 percent of cancer patients adequately comply with their doctors' instructions. If you're not doing exactly what the doctor advised, you need to ask yourself, "Why?" Perhaps your answer is a point of discussion in a conversation that should take place between you and your doctor—right away. Otherwise, you'd better be prepared to accept the risks—and possible consequences—of not following instructions that are key to your treatment or recovery.

# Part Two

# Knowing Your Options

## Chapter 4

# Getting a Second Opinion—
# and Maybe a Third

*Six months ago, a small mass appeared on a CT scan in my lung. My TWC "education" kicked in, and I was not satisfied to watch it for a year, as suggested by my oncologist. Having to pursue four doctors before being able to have a biopsy, it was finally done, and the results came back as pancreatic*

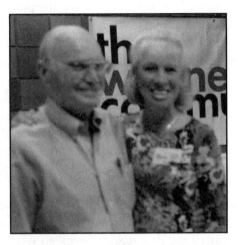

*cancer. Had I waited and not been Patient Active, the end result could have been fatal. I am doing well and again show no evidence of disease.*

—KAY KAYS,
*participant and four-time, twelve-year survivor of pancreatic cancer, The Wellness Community - Central Arizona*

OST CANCERS ARE BEST treated when they are diagnosed early. There are many types of cancer, so it's crucial that your cancer be diagnosed accurately and promptly. Treatment options depend upon careful identification of the type and stage of your cancer.

Because a *biopsy* is key to the diagnosis, it's important that you receive the appropriate type of biopsy, and that the tissue sample is evaluated by a pathologist (a doctor who specializes in studying disease through the evaluation of body tissue). Preferably, this pathologist should specialize in analyzing cancer samples. You may also need to seek out a clinical cancer center or an academic medical center to ensure that you have access to a qualified pathologist, especially if your local doctor or hospital doesn't see many cancer patients.

Feeling confident that you are receiving the best treatment for your cancer is vitally important. Even if you have good communication with your physician and are comfortable with his or her qualifications, it's often useful to seek a second—or even third—opinion at various points along the way to be certain that you are being offered the best medical treatment possible.

Keep in mind that some insurance programs even require second opinions, and many will cover such a cost if the patient requests one.

Most doctors expect and understand that because of the seriousness of cancer, patients will seek a second opinion. Don't be afraid that you will hurt your doctor's feelings, or that he or she will treat you differently. A good doctor will be respectful of your need to confirm that you are getting the best available treatment.

Consider having your consultation in a multidisciplinary setting at a major cancer center or university hospital, if possible. Some particular times you may want to seek another opinion are:

- If you've been told there is no hope and no further treatment that can be of benefit
- If there's something equivocal about your case, such as whether a tumor is operable
- If you live in a rural area and are getting treatment at a small hospital
- If you're on a managed care plan that you feel is limiting your treatment options
- If you just want to be sure you're on the right course

Your doctor will appreciate that in seeking another qualified opinion, you're gathering vital information that will help you both make even more informed decisions about your treatment.

*After giving me the names of every prominent doctor and cancer facility in many areas, [my doctor] added his own advice: 'You don't need a boob, and Tammy [my daughter] needs a mom.' My decision was made at that very moment, and I have never regretted it. I will be eternally grateful to Dr. Mastroianni.*

—LORRAINE TWARDOWSKI,
*participant, The Wellness Community - Delaware*

## Finding a Specialist

Cancer is a complex and tricky disease. The way of classifying and treating cancer can change quickly. Oncologists are doctors who specialize in cancer, and hematologists are doctors who specialize in treating disorders of the blood, including cancers such as lymphoma and leukemia.

Some specialists have a particular focus on the diagnosis and treatment of a specific type of cancer. You'll probably want to seek care from a specialist who is a member of a professional society, such as the American Society of Clinical Oncology (ASCO) or the American Association for Cancer Research (AACR). These organizations are dedicated to preventing, improving the treatment of, and curing cancer. A specialist will most likely be on the cutting edge of cancer care by reading articles and attending scientific meetings about the newest treatments for cancer.

Many oncologists are associated with a tumor board, a group made up of several kinds of cancer specialists who have different experience and backgrounds. At a tumor board meeting, a doctor can present information about you and your disease, and the other doctors will then be able to offer their opinions and ideas. However, you may prefer to get the opinion of a different oncologist, one not affiliated with the one who made the primary diagnosis. Consider having your second or third cancer consultation in a multidisciplinary setting at a major cancer center or university hospital, if possible.

Your primary doctor or your insurance company can often recommend another oncologist or cancer specialist whom you can visit to get a second opinion. If you do seek another doctor's opinion, remember that it's best to have a complete copy of your medical records, including original X-rays, pathology slides, scans, and medical reports.

It's best to get copies of all of these materials and deliver them yourself. A second opinion is not considered adequate unless another pathologist, again, preferably a cancer expert, reviews the tissue sample of the tumor itself. You might bring a friend or family member to the appointment to help take notes, ask questions, or provide support. Also, you may want to bring a tape recorder and ask the doctor if you can tape the conversation.

## Making Sense of the Numbers

The effectiveness of treatment can be seen "in the numbers," meaning statistics. But be wary of letting statistics distress you and rule your life. Remember, you're more than a number—and people aren't statistics. Those you're likely reading are merely numbers based on the experiences of large populations of people; your experience with cancer is unique and may vary greatly from the statistics.

Cancer survival statistics are based on five-year survival rates. Five-year survival can and does happen for many people with all stages of many types of cancer. You have the best odds for long-term survival if you're diagnosed with early-stage disease. Unfortunately, as the stage increases, the chance of long-term survival is reduced. However, many new treatments make it possible to manage or even control certain types of cancer for a long period of time—another good reason to seek out several medical opinions.

## Dealing with Conflicting Advice

If you receive a recommendation that's different from your original treatment plan, you'll most likely be confused. You should discuss why a different treatment plan is being proposed with both this doctor and your original doctor. For some types of cancer, there may be a multitude of treatment options, many of which are equally effective. Only you and your doctor can decide what will be the best for you. You may even feel that you need a third opinion. Because so much is at stake, it's important that you ask questions and fully discuss your medical care so that you can make the decision that is best for you.

Remember, getting a second or third opinion does not mean that you have to change your treatment course or find a new doctor. Use the information to discuss what treatment options are right for you with your initial oncologist. Many people with cancer have shared that they feel better and more in control after they've talked to another expert about their disease. As they proceed with treatment, they feel more confident that they've explored every possible option to receive the best available care.

## No "Magic Cure"

Keep in mind that going from doctor to doctor searching for a "magic cure" is not necessarily productive for your disease or your mental health. Some patients make it even harder on themselves by getting opinion after opinion, and then feeling immobilized because they can't figure out what to do. If that's happening to you or someone you know, talk to your physician, an oncology social worker, or a nurse to explore some of the fears and anxieties that you may have about making decisions about starting or ending treatment or about finding the right treatment team for you.

In some cases, you may not be able to hear what you want to hear, no matter how many doctors you go see. Be wary of any person who offers a quick or easy "cure" that doesn't seem consistent with any of the other medical professionals with whom you've discussed your case or treatment plan.

> *I went into shock with the diagnosis of pancreatic cancer. I hadn't felt bad for very long—maybe a month. I was very fortunate with the oncologist I got out of the blue. My son and daughter-in-law flew down and were here with me for my first two chemo treatments. They really liked the doctor and are now on a first-name basis with her. She's very understanding and will listen.*
>
> —BERYL LEFENER,
> *participant, The Wellness Community - Orange County*

---

**The Patient Active Doctor Interview**

Whether this is for a first, second, or third opinion, here are some great questions to ask the doctors involved in your cancer diagnosis and/or treatment:

- How much experience does he/she have in cancer and in treating cancer?
- Specifically, is he/she board certified as an oncologist, hematologist, or both?
- How does he/she stay up-to-date on the latest cancer treatments?
- Are cancer clinical trials offered at this clinic/hospital?

- What kind of radiation and surgical services are available at this clinic?
- Is the doctor or clinic associated with a major medical center, medical school, or comprehensive cancer center?
- Will this physician and/or hospital accept your type of insurance?
- Of which professional organizations is the doctor a member?
- Is there an oncology nurse or social worker that would be available during your treatment for education and support?
- What other support services (support groups, housing, etc.) are available at this clinic for patients and families?

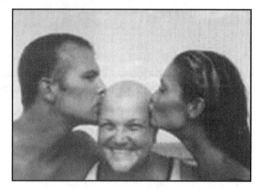

*During the past eight years, I've learned to trust my instincts, realized that seeking a second opinion can be crucial for one's survival, fine-tuned my ability to navigate the medical system, assembled a 'Multidisciplinary Medical Dream Team,' and discovered the importance of being Patient Active. Each time I've faced cancer, the more I see how essential it is for me to be a key player in the decision-making process regarding the 'action plan' for survival. Having my questions answered, along with access to up-to-date information and the pros and cons of different treatment protocols, not only decreased my anxiety level, it also empowered me to make informed decisions each step of the way.*

—BECKY GORDON,
*participant, The Wellness Community - Delmarva*

## Communicate with Your Healthcare Team

Finding out that you have cancer can be frightening and overwhelming. It can make talking (and listening!) to your doctor, nurse, other members of your healthcare team, and even your family very difficult. Fortunately, there are several things you can do to make communicating with your doctor easier. Studies show that clear communication between you and your healthcare team can help you feel better about your choices and may even improve the quality of your care.

Make sure that you understand what is being discussed. When you talk with your doctor, use "I" statements. For example, the phrase "I don't understand..." is much more effective than "You're being unclear about..." Also, be assertive. If you don't understand a word or a treatment option, say so. Make your questions specific and brief. If there's something you don't understand, ask your doctor to discuss it in more detail. Write down your questions and concerns.

Finally, if something seems confusing, try repeating it back to your doctor in this way: "You mean I should..." If you think you'll understand better with pictures, ask to see X-rays or slides, or have the doctor draw a diagram.

In order to ensure that you are getting the absolute best care and treatment, you need to be as actively involved with your healthcare team as possible. Taking all of the best information from all of the best medical minds can go a long way toward a more positive and successful outcome.

> *My oncologist, Dr. Lowell Anthony, introduced me to the surgeon who would save my life—Dr. Phil Boudreaux. His is an aggressive approach to surgery that includes excising tumors from the liver and surrounding organs. It didn't take long for me to decide. As risky as it was, at least I knew I was doing everything I could. On January 8, 2001—after nine hours of surgery—I was pronounced 85 percent cancer free. The tumors they couldn't remove were 'cooked' with radio-ablation therapy. It's been a long road back...this past winter I knew that cancer was growing again. Last March, Dr. Boudreaux and his team performed a difficult— but flawless—second surgery.*
>
> —RALPH WARRINGTON,
> *participant, The Wellness Community - Southwest Florida*

**Patient Action Plan**
- Always seek out at least one second opinion regarding your cancer diagnosis or treatment
- Forward all of your recent medical records, including operative reports, pathology reports, and radiology reports, to the outside physician with whom you'll be consulting. Call before your appointment to make sure the physician's office has received all of the necessary information prior to your visit
- Bring your original pathology slides and all of your recent radiology films, including X-rays, CT scans, MRI scans, and ultrasounds, to the appointment if they were performed at another location. Ask if you should arrive early or drop the films and slides off prior to your appointment for review
- Bring a family member or close friend to the appointment to take notes, help ask questions, and provide you with emotional support
- Consider bringing a tape recorder and asking permission to tape the conversation with your physician so that you can review the details of the consultation
- Remember, though there may not be a "magic cure" for your cancer, you'll gain the best possible benefits from the input of many experienced and knowledgeable physicians

## Chapter 5

# Traditional Treatment Options

*Years ago, before my first cancer diagnosis, I dreaded ever getting hit with the information that I had breast cancer. After my first experience, which was a lumpectomy and radiation, I found that I was able to basically return to my normal life. That which I had feared was survivable.*

—Nancy Hutchins, *participant, The Wellness Community - Central New Jersey*

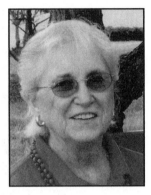

REATMENT FOR ALL TYPES of cancer is constantly evolving, but the decisions that need to be made regarding your treatment are ultimately yours to make in partnership with your healthcare team.

Most importantly, while many treatment options have similar statistics about the potential outcome, the side effects can vary widely from treatment to treatment. Therefore, not only should you talk to your doctor about the various treatment options available to you from an outcome perspective, but you should also discuss the side effects that may accompany each option and which are most acceptable for your lifestyle and goals of therapy. No one is more qualified than you to make decisions about your quality of life and your future. Seek information and advice, and then do what is right for you.

It may be important for you to talk to one or more oncology specialists: a surgeon, a medical oncologist, or a radiation oncologist. Seek advice for the most up-to-date and appropriate treatment available for your cancer. Ask your doctor about clinical trials before you make any decision about your treatment.

Remember, being Patient Active is especially critical in the *treatment* phase of your cancer experience. Therefore, you should learn as much as possible about all of the traditional treatment options available to you, while also looking at newer treatment options.

## Chemotherapy

Chemotherapy is the use of drugs to destroy cancer cells. Chemotherapeutic drugs affect rapidly growing cells—cancer and some normal cells. Because these drugs affect the cells in our bodies, we can potentially experience side effects such as hair loss, mouth sores, and risk of infection. Many side effects are temporary and cease once treatment has been completed or stopped. However, some side effects might cause physical and emotional distress that can be disruptive to the dose and frequency of chemotherapy you need to receive to have an optimal chance for recovery.

The type of chemotherapy given depends on the type of cancer, the stage of your cancer, and your overall health. More than half of the people diagnosed with cancer get chemotherapy. There are many different types of "chemo" drugs available, but, generally, you and your oncologist will discuss a specific protocol or treatment plan that is considered the standard of care for your cancer in its present form.

One of the most critical things you need to consider with chemotherapy is that it's important to "stay the course." Unnecessary changes or delays in your chemotherapy treatment schedule can have physical and emotional consequences. It's very important that you report all symptoms or side effects to your doctor and/or nurse so that they can be treated effectively.

### Dose Intensity Is Key

In one recent study, an ongoing review of medical charts for more than 17,000 women with early-stage breast cancer receiving chemotherapy showed that:

- Up to 20 percent of patients were receiving less than 85 percent of the planned chemotherapy dose intensity. Data suggests that dose intensity above 85 percent may result in a better chance for relapse-free and overall survival

- Twenty-eight percent of these women had their chemotherapy doses lowered. Forty-four percent had to have treatments rescheduled

## Not Your Grandmother's Chemotherapy

Many of the stories you may have heard about chemotherapy treatments are no longer true. More effective drugs in higher doses and different combinations that improve the possibility of long-term survivorship—at least for certain cancers—have been developed. Modern advances in medications that reduce—or completely eliminate—nausea and vomiting, as well as cancer pain, have been made. Other special medications, called blood cell growth factors, are available to help your blood counts return to normal more quickly. This reduces the possibility of infection and unnecessary hospitalizations.

Chemotherapy is generally administered in the outpatient clinic on a regular schedule for a specified period of time. You may receive a combination or sequence of drugs proven to be most effective. Chemotherapy may be given *intravenously* (by vein), in pill form (by mouth), through an injection (shot), or applied directly on the skin. You need to get extensive information from your doctor and oncology nurse as to what specific treatment you'll need and what to expect in the weeks and months ahead. You may want to chart out your treatment schedule and follow-up appointments on a special calendar so you can stay on schedule.

*I remember meeting with the surgeon, who held up the X-rays and said, 'That's cancer,' pointing to one of the spots, not being sure of the others. Now, we started to talk about needle biopsies versus surgical biopsies and realized this was only the first of many decisions we would need to make on our journey. We* 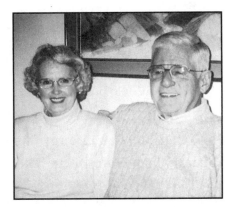 *added new words to our everyday vocabulary—words like 'HER-2,' 'estrogen receptors,' 'mastectomies,' 'chemotherapy,' 'adriamycin,' and 'radiation.'*

—ROBERT LUBRECHT,
*participant, The Wellness Community -
Greater Cincinnati/Northern Kentucky*

## How Does Chemotherapy Work?

Normal cells grow and die in a controlled way. When cancer occurs, cells in the body that are not normal keep dividing and forming more cells out of control. Chemotherapy drugs destroy cancer cells by stopping them from growing and multiplying. Healthy cells can also be harmed, especially those that divide quickly. Harm to the healthy cells is what causes side effects. The kind of side effects you may experience depends on the kind of chemotherapy drugs you are getting, the dosages, and the frequency of treatments. Previously healthy cells usually repair themselves after chemotherapy, but it's important that you actively manage any side effects you may experience.

### Goals of Chemotherapy
Depending on the type of cancer and how advanced it is, chemotherapy can be used for different goals:
- **To cure the cancer**.
    Cancer is considered cured when the patient remains free of any evidence of measurable tumor on physical examination or laboratory and radiology studies
- **To control the cancer**.
    Control is keeping the cancer from spreading, slowing the cancer's growth, and killing cancer cells that may have spread to other parts of the body from the original tumor
- **To relieve symptoms that the cancer may be causing**.
    Relieving symptoms such as pain and discomfort can help patients live more comfortably

## How Can You Prepare for Chemotherapy?

Patients who prepare for chemotherapy say they are better able to handle the physical and emotional effects of the treatment. Talk to others who've been through the experience.

- Talk to your physician, and carefully weigh the many options presented to you
- Set goals and rewards for yourself as you reach treatment milestones
- Pray and seek spiritual support
- Be active in gathering information and getting second opinions
- Prepare a question list, and keep a journal of your visits with the doctor
- Tape-record the conversation with the doctor to play again for yourself or family members
- Bring someone with you for emotional support and to hear what's being said so you can discuss it together later
- Talk to your oncology nurse about your questions or concerns
- Consider talking to a social worker or counselor to help you and your family prepare for emotional and social issues
- Join a support group with others who are going through cancer treatment
- Anticipate certain physical side effects such as *fatigue*, hair loss, nausea, fever, and infection

## Radiation Treatment

Radiation treatment is the use of high-energy X-rays to stop cancer cells from growing and multiplying. Also referred to as radiotherapy, X-ray, cobalt, or irradiation therapy, radiation therapy is usually given to the exterior of your body by a machine that can pinpoint high-energy beams directly to the location of your cancer. Half of all people with cancer are treated with radiation. For many patients, radiation is the only kind of treatment needed.

Radiation therapy is given in doses (measured in rads or grays), usually five days a week for several weeks. You'll work very closely with the radiation oncologist and a highly skilled group of radiation technicians who will support you with high-tech, high-quality care.

Prior to radiation, you'll get precise measurements of exactly where the radiotherapy is to be given. The technicians will draw special markings on your skin to guide them—and the machine—in giving you effective treatment. You will not be radioactive during this time and generally won't feel anything during the treatment itself, except perhaps a little discomfort due to lying still for a period of time. Many people are able to arrange their daily radiation appointments around work or other daily activities. Sometimes the best time to go is early in the morning; that way, you have your whole day to be active.

Another kind of radiation treatment involves internal radiation: an exact amount of radioactive material, implanted inside your body, usually in an area that involves cancer of the vagina, prostate, or breast. The implant is left there for a few days. During that time, you'll generally stay in the hospital while the radioactive implant works to destroy the tumor.

> **Goals of Radiation Therapy**
> Like chemotherapy, the goal of radiotherapy depends on the type of cancer and how advanced it is. Radiotherapy can be used to:
> - **Shrink the tumor.**
>     Radiation can be an important tool to stop the growth of cancer cells that remain after surgery or to reduce the size of a tumor before surgery
> - **Improve quality of life.**
>     Even when curing the cancer isn't possible, radiation therapy can still bring relief. Many patients find that symptoms, such as pain, are greatly improved with radiotherapy

*Doctors do half the work in healing, and we have to do the other half: healing emotions and spirit.*

—DIANA BERHO,
*participant, The Wellness Community - South Bay Cities*

## Surgery

Surgery can be used in the diagnosis, staging, and treatment of cancer. It can also be used to minimize the symptoms of advanced disease and to relieve distress, or for reconstructive and rehabilitative purposes. Many people have a biopsy to confirm or diagnose cancer correctly. A biopsy consists of extracting a tissue sample from an organ or other part of the body for examination by a pathologist. A positive biopsy indicates the presence of cancer, whereas a negative biopsy may indicate that no cancer was present or that the biopsy specimen was inadequate. Surgery has played a major role in the cure of melanoma, breast, colorectal, and thyroid cancers—if caught early.

A common unproven myth is that surgery may cause cancer to spread by exposing the cancerous cells to air. This just isn't true. Cancer doesn't spread because it's been exposed to air. However, some patients feel worse after surgery than they did before it due to discomfort from the incision and anesthesia. This feeling is absolutely normal. Because early removal of all cancer cells provides the best chance of a cure, it's important that you not allow this myth to discourage you from seeking surgery.

> **Goals of Surgery**
> - **Diagnose and stage the cancer**.
>   Surgery can identify the tumor type, extent of growth, size nodal involvement, and regional and/or distant spread
> - **Cure**.
>   The primary goal of cancer surgery is to cure. Definitive or curative surgery involves removing the entire tumor, associated lymph nodes, and a two- to five-centimeter margin of surrounding tissue. To increase the likelihood of a cure, early detection is essential
> - **Relieve symptoms**.
>   Surgery can be used to minimize symptoms of advanced disease, such as neurosurgical procedures for pain control
> - **Reconstruct or rehabilitate**.
>   The goal is to minimize deformity and improve quality of life (as in breast, head, and neck reconstruction)

## Should a Surgeon Say, "I Got It All?"

In general, when a surgeon says, "I got it all," it means that the tumor was removed in its entirety, the margins (area around the tumor) were clean and free of cancer cells, and there was no evidence of lymph node or metastatic spread. Because approximately 70 percent of patients have evidence of micrometastases at the time of diagnosis, this statement should be made with extreme caution. It may be less misleading to the patient if the surgeon says, "Apparently there is no evidence of cancer left behind. In a couple of days, we'll have a pathology report that'll give us more information. If the pathology is clear at the margins, there's a good chance that it's all been removed." However, there's still a chance that microscopic disease has already spread. That's why it's important to see an oncologist to talk about additional therapies such as chemotherapy and/or radiation therapy.

Surgery alone can be curative in patients with localized disease, but it's often necessary to combine surgery with other treatment modalities in order to achieve higher response rates.

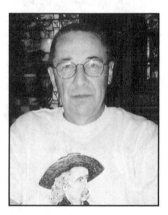

*During my recovery from surgery, I found great consolation in trips to a local botanical garden and to the art museum in town. I also let my church know that I had cancer—but not that it was terminal—and received great support from my friends and pastor.*

—STEVE AHLF,
*participant, The Wellness Community - Greater St. Louis*

**The Wellness Community Treatment Decision-Making Tool**
This tool is designed to help you discuss treatment options with your doctor.
Bring it to your appointment and use it as a guide as you make decisions about the right treatment for you.

**PART ONE**

| Medical Background Questions | Answers |
| --- | --- |
| When was I diagnosed?<br>(A person with newly diagnosed cancer may have different treatment options than a person who has already had certain treatments.) | |
| What type of cancer do I have?<br>(The type of cancer will determine the type of treatment you need.) | |
| What is the stage of my cancer?<br>(The stage of the cancer will also determine the types of treatments available.) | |
| What is my current health status?<br>(Your overall health status may affect the types of treatments you can tolerate.) | |
| What should be the goal of my treatment?<br>(The goal of treatment—cure, symptom control, prolonged remission—may affect the type of treatment that is available to you or that you select.) | |

**PART TWO**

| Treatment Options | As you discuss treatment options with your doctor, take notes under each column below. | | |
|---|---|---|---|
| YOU HAVE CHOICES! | Potential Side Effects (i.e., hospitalization, hair loss, fatigue, peripheral neuropathy, nausea and vomiting, rash, etc.) | Quality of Life/ Treatment Convenience (i.e, required visits to the hospital or clinic to receive treatment, monitoring, blood counts, restricting activities, etc.) | Effectiveness (i.e., what are the chances that this treatment will work for me?) |
| Surgery (Can the tumor be surgically removed?) | | | |
| Pre- or Post-Surgery Chemotherapy | | | |
| Pre- or Post-Surgery Radiation | | | |
| Radiation | | | |
| Chemotherapy | | | |
| Novel Therapies | | | |
| Investigational Therapies in Clinical Trials | | | |
| Combination Treatments (from above) | | | |
| Best Supportive Care | | | |

**Patient Action Plan**

- Talk to your physician, and carefully weigh the many options presented to you
- Set goals and rewards for yourself as you reach treatment milestones
- Pray, and seek spiritual support
- Be active in gathering information and getting second opinions
- Prepare a question list, and keep a journal of your visits with the doctor
- Tape-record the conversation with the doctor to play again for yourself or family members
- Bring someone with you for emotional support and to hear what's being said so you can discuss it together later
- Talk to your oncology nurse about your questions or concerns
- Consider talking to a social worker or counselor to help you and your family prepare for emotional and social issues
- Join a support group with others who are going through cancer treatment
- Anticipate certain physical side effects such as fatigue, hair loss, nausea, fever, and infection
- Remember that you always have choices

## Chapter 6

# New Frontiers in Treatment

*I am more focused on my immune system and how to take care of it.*

—NAS FARSAI,
*participant, The Wellness Community - Orange County*

■ MAGINE A DOCTOR BEING able to identify the best treatment for you personally—just by studying a tissue sample and cataloging your genetic make-up or by being able to have a treatment that attacks the precise sections of a cell that causes it to grow into a tumor. While these scenarios are still imaginary today, the progress of science and medicine could make these realistic situations in the near future.

Advances are being made in the understanding of how cancer occurs, how to treat it, and ultimately how to prevent it. It's not easy; cancer includes more than 100 different diseases, but there's definitely hope. Everyday, scientists are uncovering new discoveries such as *apoptosis*, chemotherapy combinations, *cancer vaccines*, biologic and gene therapy, and other new technologies.

## Starting at the Cellular Level

It's widely known today that early detection of cancer can dramatically increase the rate of survival. Along with treatment advances, another branch of cancer research involves finding new tools to diagnose the disease. These new tools help detect cancer earlier, determine the stages of the disease, monitor the progression of cancer, and select the most effective therapies. Current research is concentrating on cellular and gene-based testing to help accomplish these goals.

Some cellular tests are being used to detect and count circulating tumor cells (CTCs) in a blood sample. Gene-based testing (also called molecular testing) determines the presence and tissue origin of cancer cells to establish disease staging and will most likely help in prognostic and therapy selection. Molecular tests offer the potential for greater accuracy and more patient-specific information. Many tests are still in the investigative phase and have not yet been approved for widespread use. At The Wellness Community, we hope that someday a test will be discovered that not only detects cancer once it occurs, but that also detects it as a precancerous condition from its start—at the very earliest cellular level.

## New Treatment Tools

One of the newest treatment tools against cancer is called *targeted therapy*. Targeted cancer therapies work differently than traditional approaches, such as radiation and chemotherapy. These treatments aim to impact tumor cells without compromising healthy cells in the process. This approach can produce fewer side effects in people undergoing treatment for cancer.

Scientific advances have shown that many of the changes in cells that lead to cancer are due to genes and something called the *signal system* within a cell. Targeted therapies work to interfere with the signal system, which either tells a cancer cell to multiply or to destroy itself. Targeted therapies are designed to interfere with cancer cell growth and division in different ways and at various points during the development, growth, and spread of cancer. Many of these therapies focus on proteins that are involved in the signaling process within and between cells. Targeted therapies work by blocking cell signals that promote cancer growth.

*It's important to note that new therapies are not always appropriate for every cancer treatment, so you should definitely talk with your doctor to find out if any of the newer treatments might be appropriate for your condition.*

The most common currently available or soon-to-be-available categories of targeted therapies include treatments that utilize the following:

- *Monoclonal antibodies* targeting cancer cell growth
- *Anti-angiogenesis drugs* targeting tumor blood vessel growth
- Small molecules: *tyrosine kinase* and *heterodimerization inhibitors*

Some of the most important targeted therapies in use or in development today include variations of therapeutic antibodies, Anti-CD 20/B cell monoclonal antibody, *Epidermal Growth Factor Receptors (EGFRs)*, and anti-angiogenesis agents (such as *vascular endothelial growth factor, or VEGF*).

## More Cancer Treatments on the Horizon

Several categories of cancer treatments are currently being investigated for the future. These include apoptosis-inducing drugs targeting cancer cell death; new combinations of targeted agents, cancer vaccines, *biologic therapy* or *immunotherapy*, and *gene therapies*.

## Therapeutic Monoclonal Antibodies

One of the newer types of therapies available today is therapeutic antibodies. To understand what therapeutic antibodies are, you must first understand how the body's *immune system* works. *Antibodies* are proteins found in the body that are made in response to foreign antigens. An *antigen* is any substance that produces a sensitivity response by the body when it comes into contact with tissue. We usually think of an antigen as anything foreign that produces a "fight" response by the body's immune system. The body produces specific antibodies to specific antigens. The antibody attaches to the antigen, and a reaction that usually results in the destruction of the antigen is triggered. This process allows for the protection of our bodies against infection and disease.

In the 1950s, scientists began to explore methods of using the body's immune system to help fight cancer. Researchers wanted to develop specific antibodies that would attach to and destroy cancer cells. It took twenty years of research to develop laboratory methods that would produce a single antibody that recognized a single antigen, or a monoclonal antibody. This method, called the *hybridoma technique*, opened the door for scientists to make unlimited amounts of pure monoclonal antibodies. By the 1980s, scientists were sure that a "magic bullet" to cure cancer would soon be discovered.

Early monoclonal antibodies were produced from mouse cells. However, a major problem developed when they were given to humans, because the body recognized the mouse proteins in the antibodies as foreign. Patients experienced severe allergic reactions as the body sought to destroy the foreign antibodies. It would take another twenty years for scientists to overcome the problems of using mouse cells to make monoclonal antibodies safe for use in humans. The monoclonal antibodies in use today are made from mouse and human proteins. There's still a risk of an allergic reaction when receiving a monoclonal antibody, but severe reactions are rare, and the potential benefit has been promising.

Several therapeutic antibodies are now in use, and many more are being studied in clinical trials. Therapeutic antibodies are the general category that includes monoclonal antibodies used to treat cancer and other diseases. They are designed to react with cancer cells in a way that triggers the body to fight a cancer more effectively, and they represent a growing family of "targeted therapies."

Monoclonal antibody therapy aims to target tumor cells that have a certain protein antigen on the surface of the cell. When a monoclonal antibody binds with the protein antigen on cancer cells, it helps the body's general immune response. The antibody acts like a key that fits only one lock (antigen) on the cell surface. Once the key is inserted into the lock, one of several actions may occur: the signals to the core of the cell (nucleus) can be blocked, so normal cell functions, such as growth and repair, do not occur; the key can attract other cells of the immune system or other blood proteins to destroy the cell; or the signal for cell death can be launched. Any of these actions can result in stopping cell function or in cell death—which is the ultimate goal for targeting cancer cells.

> *I told my Ohio doctor that I wanted Zevalin®, and he arranged for me to have the treatment. I was treated in June 2004, and as of July 2006, my scans are showing no enlarged lymph nodes. It's amazing not to need treatment for this long. I feel healthy and my blood counts are good. . . . I don't need another CAT scan until next June.*
>
> —Jan Waters,
> *participant, The Wellness Community - Greater Columbus*

## Joining Forces with Chemotherapy

Therapeutic monoclonal antibodies alone can interfere with cell functions, or they can work in partnership with agents that are attached to them to target and kill tumor cells. Examples of agents that attach to the monoclonal antibody include radiation agents, chemotherapy, or other *biologic agents*. Once the monoclonal antibody carries the other agent along to the target, the agent can direct its killing effect on the tumor cell to destroy the cancer.

*Chemotherapy* acts very differently when it's working with a monoclonal antibody than when it acts alone. Chemotherapy is non-selective, which means that it affects all cells dividing at certain phases. Because the drugs kill both normal and cancerous cells, there are body-wide (systemic) side effects. Tumor cells can develop a resistance to chemotherapy drugs over time. Monoclonal antibody therapy is more tumor-specific, but it's not perfect. The monoclonal antibody targets a specific antigen on the surface of the tumor cell. Normal, healthy cells are not usually affected. Therefore, when chemotherapy is delivered only to the surface of the tumor cell, the side effects can be much milder than if the chemotherapy is circulated throughout the entire body. This is a real milestone in new discoveries for cancer because it may increasingly help doctors find a way to identify specific cells in your body that are receptive to certain cancer treatments—thereby directly targeting the cancer cells for destruction and reducing the impact of unwanted side effects or resistance.

## Currently Used Therapeutic Monoclonal Antibodies

Right now, therapeutic monoclonal antibodies being used in cancer treatment include: anti-CD 20/B cell, *anti-EGFR*, and anti-angiogenesis. Let's take a closer look at each.

## Anti-CD 20/B Cell Monoclonal Antibodies

Scientists have discovered that people with non-Hodgkin's lymphoma (NHL) have a specific antigen (lock) on the cell surface called CD 20. In normal cells, the CD 20 antigen helps in the growth and maturation of one type of lymphocyte called *B-lymphocytes*, which help in the immune system. CD 20 antigens also play a role in helping tumor cell growth. A number of newly developed treatments target the CD 20 antigen to stop the growth of the cancer.

A specific anti-CD 20/B cell monoclonal antibody, *Rituxan®* (*rituximab*), was developed to attach to the CD 20 antigen on normal and malignant B-cells, where they recruit the body's natural defenses to attack and kill the marked B-cells. The CD 20 antigen is not present during the early development of B-cells. Therefore, with Rituxan, B-cells can *regenerate* after treatment and return to their normal functions. Rituxan has been approved by the FDA as a single-agent treatment in patients with relapsed or refractory, low-grade or follicular (indolent) non-Hodgkin's lymphoma. It is also approved as a single-agent treatment in patients who have shown a partial or complete response to earlier chemotherapy. In combination with chemotherapy, Rituxan is approved by the FDA as part of a first-line treatment regimen for patients with untreated indolent or untreated diffuse large cell non-Hodgkin's lymphoma. It is also used for other diseases, such as chronic lymphocytic leukemia (CLL) or Waldenstrom's macroglobulinemia.

It's generally administered as an *IV infusion* once a week for four or eight doses. There are side effects, such as infusion reactions and infection. It's important to review the possible side effects and precautions with your doctor if you're considering this or any of the other options discussed here.

Another type of monoclonal antibody is used in conjunction with a *radioactive isotope* (*radioisotope*) in a type of treatment that is called *radioimmunotherapy* (*RIT*). *Zevalin®* (*ibritumomab tiuxetan*) is an FDA-approved radioimmunotherapy treatment that also targets the CD 20 antigen found on B-cell non-Hodgkin's lymphoma patients. The monoclonal antibody has a radioisotope attached to it that delivers radiation therapy to the lymphoma cells; however, this indication is only for relapsed/refractory non-Hodgkin's lymphoma and for patients who are refractory to Rituxan. The Zevalin therapeutic regimen consists of yttrium-90 labeled ibritumomab tiuxetal and unlabeled rituximab; in this treatment regimen, Zevalin is not used alone. With this dual-action therapy, cancer cells are destroyed by both high-energy radiation and the cell-killing action of the monoclonal antibody. When used in non-Hodgkin's lymphoma, radio-labeled monoclonal antibodies target specific cells and destroy cancer cells, while minimizing damage to normal cells. Side effects include risk of infection, fatigue due to *anemia*, and bleeding.

The most recently approved targeted radioimmunotherapy treatment is *Bexxar®*, which is made of two parts: a monoclonal antibody named *tositumomab* and a monoclonal antibody with radiation attached named *iodine-131 tositumomab*. This two-part treatment is used in patients with *CD 20 positive*, non-Hodgkin's lymphoma whose disease is no longer responding to Rituxan and has relapsed after chemotherapy.

The unlabeled tositumomab portion of the agent with no radiation attached binds to the tumor cells and attracts other cells of the immune system, such as *T-lymphocytes*, which then attack the tumor cell. The labeled tositumomab portion with I-131 (the attached radiation) also locks on to other lymphoma cells and delivers a low, continuous dose of radiation directly to the cancer cells. This therapy is a little more complex to administer, and patients are given medications up front to limit side effects and prevent damage to the thyroid gland by the radiation. Other side effects are similar to those already mentioned.

## Anti-EGFR Monoclonal Antibodies

Another type of monoclonal antibody currently in use is called *anti-EGFRs*. There is a family of *receptors* found on the surface of normal and cancer cells called *Human Epidermal Growth Factor Receptors (EGFR)*. Something called an *epidermal growth factor* binds to these receptor proteins, causing the cells to divide.

In healthy cells, an amount of this protein on the cell surface reacts with the growth factors that come along and cell division remains within normal limits. The problem comes when there are abnormally high levels of this receptor protein on the cell surface, such as in many types of cancer cells, which scientists believe may be partly responsible for the fact that cancer cells divide and multiply uncontrollably. Specific tests can measure whether the amount of the EGFR protein on the cancer cells is abnormally high. This can affect the kind of treatment that is recommended for the person with cancer. There are at least four members of this genetic "family": *HER1*, *HER2*, *HER3*, and *HER4*.

One important member of this family, HER2, is used to identify if there is risk for excessive growth in certain cells. If the HER2 growth signal is unusually strong, or "*HER2 positive*," the nucleus tells the cell to divide and grow rapidly, which contributes to the development of a more *aggressive cancer*. Studies in cancer patients have shown that about 25–30 percent of all women with breast cancer have too many HER2 receptors. This seems to be an important reason why tumor cells grow and divide so rapidly. Knowledge of a woman's HER2 status can affect her course of treatment for breast cancer.

*Herceptin®* (*trastuzumab*) is the first monoclonal antibody created from human cells and approved by the FDA for the treatment of HER2 positive metastatic breast cancer. It has also recently been approved for the treatment of patients with early-stage disease. Herceptin works by targeting tumor cells that have too many HER2 receptors, also known as *HER2 over-expression*. When the cell signal is stopped, the cancer cells' ability to continue to grow and divide is also stopped. This process is unique because only cells with HER2 over-expression are targeted by Herceptin. Standard chemotherapy kills cells that are dividing, which means that both breast cancer cells and normal cells are destroyed. This causes many of the side effects associated with chemotherapy, such as hair loss, nausea and vomiting, and risk of infection and bleeding. Because Herceptin interferes with the cell signaling in only the breast cancer cells, there are fewer side effects. However, some problems with cardiac toxicity may prevent some patients from receiving this antibody.

Herceptin is approved for women with breast cancer:

- For *first-line* (first treatment after diagnosis) use in combination with a chemotherapy drug called *Taxol®* (*paclitaxel*)
- As a single agent (used alone) in second- and third-line treatment after the breast cancer has recurred

In combination with doxorubicin, cyclophosphamide, and paclitaxel for treatment after surgery to remove the tumor of patients with early-stage breast cancer, thousands of women have had a good response to this drug, and their cancer has reduced in size or disappeared. It's still unknown precisely how long the drug should be given, so research is ongoing. Herceptin has become a landmark biologic therapy for women with HER2 over-expressive metastatic cancer.

There are two approved tests to determine if a woman shows HER2 positive status with metastatic breast cancer:

- *FISH* (*fluorescence in situ hybridization*) measures with fluorescent dye the number of genes in each cell of a tissue sample to test for HER2 status. FISH uses a probe that marks its matching DNA in the cell nucleus with a fluorescent tag. If more than two fluorescent signals for HER2 are seen, it shows that an increase of HER2 receptors on the surface of the cell has occurred

- *IHC (immunohistochemistry)* also tests a tissue sample by using specific antibodies that recognize and stain cell-surface receptors. The antibodies bind to the receptors and make it possible to detect the number and location of HER2 receptors that are present in the cell. If an abnormally large number of cell-surface receptors are seen, over-expression has occurred

Erbitux (cetuximab) and Vectibix (panitumumab) are two new anti-EGFR monoclonal anti-body treatments targeting a different member of the EGFR family: the HER1 receptor, which is also called EGFR. In clinical trials, this monoclonal antibody has been found to bind with the HER1 or EGFR receptor to stop cell growth signals in people with colon cancer. It's been discovered that many people with colon cancer have EGFR over-expression, in which too many EGFR or HER1 receptors are found on the cell surface. When Erbitux binds with the receptor, the EGFR can no longer cause the tumor cells to grow and divide. Erbitux alone (intravenously) or in combination with radiation therapy is also approved by the FDA for the treatment of advanced head and neck cancer.

There is one test, immunohistochemistry (IHC), to determine if a person with metastatic colon cancer shows an over-expression of EGFR or HER1 receptors. IHC is done on a tumor tissue sample taken at the time of surgery or biopsy, which determines if the colon cancer cells show EGFR positive status.

Both of the anti-EGFR monoclonal antibodies listed here, Herceptin and Erbitux, can be given safely. However, infusion reactions can occur (i.e., fever, chills, nausea), especially during the first treatment. There are also new side effects, such as an acne-like rash, weakness, and diarrhea. Many of these side effects can be lessened with other medications. (*For more information on side effects, see Chapter 9.*)

## Anti-Angiogenesis Monoclonal Antibodies

*Angiogenesis* is a normal biologic process in which new blood vessels grow from existing healthy cells. During the development and spread of cancer, this process works against the body when it is "turned on" by tumors to feed their growth. New blood vessels may "feed" cancer cells with oxygen and nutrients, allowing the cells to grow, move into nearby tissue, and spread to other parts of the body.

This important finding, discovered in the 1980s, is enabling scientists to have a better understanding of how tumor cells feed themselves and grow. Therefore, it helps scientists determine ways to reverse or stop this process. Selectively stopping the process of angiogenesis by cutting off, or "starving," the support system of tumor cells is called *anti-angiogenesis*. Anti-angiogenesis is a way to stop new blood vessels from growing in tumor cells, thereby "starving" and eventually killing the tumor cells.

In order to stimulate anti-angiogenesis in tumor cells, scientists found the important target: Vascular Endothelial Growth Factor. VEGF is a protein or growth factor involved in the process of angiogenesis. VEGF stimulates growth and is necessary for production of the blood vessels that transport nutrients and oxygen to cells and organs. Without these vessels, tumors have difficulty growing. VEGF is produced naturally by the body but can also be produced in abnormal amounts by certain tumor cells, such as colorectal cancer cells. An increased amount of VEGF in the bloodstream has been linked with a poor outcome, or *prognosis*, in colorectal cancer.

Here's an analogy: If a car were able to make its own gasoline, it would drive forever. In this case, the gasoline for the cancer cell is VEGF, which is made by the cancer cell itself. When the car (cancer cell) can no longer use gasoline (VEGF) to feed itself, it breaks down (the cancer cell dies).

*Avastin®* (*bevacizumab*), a unique drug that has recently been approved by the FDA, is modeled on this process. Avastin is approved for use in the *first- or second-line treatment* of metastatic colorectal cancer, in combination with chemotherapy (5-flourouracil). Avastin in combination with carboplatin and paclitaxel chemotherapy has also recently been approved for the treatment of advanced non-small cell lung cancer. When VEGF is joined with the monoclonal antibody, it can no longer bind with the receptor site, and blood vessels cannot grow, causing the tumor to "starve." Therefore, it stops the cancer cells from feeding themselves, to the point where the colon cancer cells die. When combining this targeted approach with chemotherapy, there are fewer additional side effects than with some of the more traditional treatments for metastatic colon cancer. Avastin is also being evaluated in renal cell cancer and metastatic breast cancer.

Avastin is given intravenously every two to three weeks and continues until there's no sign of disease. There are fewer infusion reactions with this monoclonal antibody than the others already mentioned.

Therefore, no medications are needed before the infusion except for those given with the chemotherapy. Because Avastin interferes with new blood cell production, it shouldn't be given to patients who are having surgery, as it may interfere with normal healing processes. High blood pressure may occur, but it can be easily managed with drugs that lower blood pressure. The risk of *bowel perforation* is also possible. Patients using this treatment should report any side effects to their doctor immediately.

The treatment of metastatic colorectal cancer has changed dramatically with the addition of the three new monoclonal antibodies, Erbitux, Vectibix, and Avastin. Research continues to determine how long the drugs can be given and whether they can be used in the treatment of early-stage colorectal cancer to prevent the spread or recurrence of the disease.

## Small Molecules, Big Effect

Another new discovery in the treatment of cancer is the development of a class of small molecules, or tyrosine kinase inhibitors (TKIs), as well as small molecule inhibitors of angiogenesis, such as Sutent (sunitinib) and Nexavar (sorafenib). Both drugs are approved for renal cell carcinoma; Sutent is also approved for a rare form of stomach cancer called gastrointestinal stromal tumor (GIST). The tyrosine kinase (TK) area of a cell is in charge of allowing cells to divide and multiply. During normal cell activity, the receptor of a cell, found on the outer portion of the cell, receives the growth factor. The receptor then sends a signal that goes inside of the cell into the TK area. Here, chemical actions occur, and the signal is sent along one or more pathways to the nucleus (center, or brain) of the cell, where the cell is told to multiply.

Tyrosine kinase inhibitors are made of small molecules that allow them easily to enter the tumor cell and attach to the TK area, which is found within the epidermal growth factor receptor. While inside this area, TKIs actually stop the signal from getting to the nucleus of the tumor cell and, therefore, stop the cell from multiplying.

*Gleevec® (imatinib mesylate)* is the first FDA-approved drug that directly turns off the signal of a protein known to cause a cancer. Since its debut in 2001, Gleevec has been hailed as a "miracle" cancer treatment that works by blocking an abnormal enzyme found on the tumor cells. Unfortunately, doctors have discovered that, over time, some patients can develop a resistance to the drug, and it becomes less effective. Nevertheless, Gleevec has become a model for developing precise treatments that stop cancer earlier in its molecular tracks.

Gleevec is indicated for adult and pediatric chronic myelogenous leukemia (CML) and a rare form of stomach cancer called gastrointestinal stromal tumor (GIST). It's also being investigated for effectiveness against other kinds of cancer.

Another TKI drug has completed Phase III clinical trials and was approved by the FDA in late 2004. *Tarceva* (*erlotinib HCl*) is a small molecule designed to block the HER1 signaling pathway of the cancer cell. It has been approved for use in patients with non-small cell lung cancer and pancreatic cancer that has recurred after standard treatment. In addition, it is being studied on other tumors, such as ovarian, colorectal, head and neck, renal cell, brain (glioma), and gastrointestinal cancers. This drug interferes with the cell growth signal by attaching to the TK portion of the EGFR. The reported side effects for this TKI are also mild-to-moderate skin rash and diarrhea.

## Heterodimerization Inhibitors (HDIs)

Understanding the epidermal growth factor receptor genes (HER1, HER2, HER3, and HER4) has also led to the new discovery that combinations of these receptors may ultimately stop cancer cell growth and survival. Each of these receptors has a role in cell growth, maturation, and survival. The signal begins with a growth factor that joins two receptors and activates them to send a signal inside the cell. When two different receptors join, the activation is called *heterodimerization*; when two of the same cells join, it's called *homodimerization*.

Because scientists are now learning that some cancers "over-express" more than one EGFR at the same time, current research is focused on finding agents that stop heterodimerization. This group of agents is called *heterodimerization inhibitors*. It's not a simple matter to stop the excess signaling by cell receptors, as there are a number of different growth factors and a number of ways the receptors can pair up. This is a fascinating new area of research for targeted cancer treatment.

One example of a drug that uses this mechanism is called *Omnitarg*™ (*pertuzumab*). Omnitarg is one of the first in a new class of targeted therapeutic agents, known as heterodimerization inhibitors (HDIs), currently being evaluated in clinical trials in the treatment of lung cancer, ovarian cancer, and prostate cancer. Omnitarg has not yet been approved by the FDA; however, Phase III clinical trials continue, in the hope of receiving a wide approval.

There are many new discoveries in cancer that may someday change how cancer is detected, treated, controlled, or even prevented. The new discoveries that are in use today include targeted therapies such as monoclonal antibodies, anti-EGFR agents, anti-angiogenesis, and the discovery of small molecules. You may want to talk with your doctor about whether any of these new discoveries might be helpful in your situation.

## Targeting Apoptosis Pathways

Scientists are also exploring the possibility of targeting certain pathways (ways that cells control their actions) that cancer cells use to grow and divide.

One pathway that is being studied is called the *apoptosis pathway*. Apoptosis is a normal process, also called "programmed cell death." It's a way for the body to naturally destroy diseased or damaged cells. Several pathways and proteins have been identified that regulate apoptosis.

Discoveries have also been made to indicate that *mutations* in cancer cells may make these apoptosis pathways ineffective. This would mean that cancer cells would no longer get a signal to die; conversely, they would be allowed to continue to grow and multiply. Proteins like TRAIL (tumor necrosis factor related apoptosis-inducing ligand) Receptor-1, also known as Apo2L, that cause apoptosis have been discovered. Clinical trials are testing drugs that would recognize and mimic these proteins and, hopefully, increase tumor cell death. This method to induce apoptosis provides another promising new approach to targeted cancer therapy.

*Another promising approach is to combine targeting agents so that they interrupt the signals that promote cancer growth at different points in the cell signaling system. This research could lead to more effective and powerful drug combinations that are less toxic and more specifically designed to destroy cancer cells in a way that would protect people from some of the side effects or relapses seen with standard chemotherapy regimens.*

## Cancer Vaccines

Therapeutic cancer vaccines are another future treatment option in development. For most of us, the word "vaccine" brings to mind a way to prevent an illness, such as the flu or polio. Cancer vaccines are different in three important ways:

- They're a new approach to help treat cancer—not prevent it. (Vaccines are being studied to prevent liver and cervical cancers, but the term "cancer vaccine" usually refers to a type of treatment)
- They're still very much in the experimental stage for many types of cancer
- They'll most likely be used along with standard treatments, rather than as a stand-alone treatment

Therapeutic cancer vaccines are available only through clinical trials, and, for now, only a small number of people can participate in them. But that may change. Scientists are exploring cancer vaccines for many cancers, including breast, colorectal, melanoma, non-Hodgkin's lymphoma, non-small cell lung, ovarian, and prostate cancer. A cervical cancer vaccine was also approved by the FDA in 2006.

## How Cancer Vaccines Work

Because cancer cells are "insiders" and have a mechanism to help make them invisible to the body's immune system, cancer cells can multiply into large tumors without triggering an effective immune response. Cancer vaccines counter these tactics by tricking the immune system into recognizing the tumor and prompting the immune system to fight back.

Cancer vaccines have several proven and potential advantages over standard therapies:

- **They are very well tolerated, with few and fairly minor side effects.**
  This is because they help the immune system distinguish if cells are tumor or normal cells, so that only harmful cells will be attacked. Standard therapy kills both tumor cells and healthy cells, causing unpleasant—and sometimes serious—side effects
- **They may produce longer remissions or prevent recurrence.**
  Once the immune system is triggered to attack tumor cells,

it may remain on alert longer to destroy them. With standard therapy, a few resistant tumor cells are often able to survive and cause a return of the disease

- **They may be effective even against metastatic disease—cancer that has spread beyond its initial site to other parts of the body.**
  The immune system serves the entire body and can hunt down and destroy wandering tumor cells wherever they gather

Though results from clinical trials are still inconclusive, some cases of reduced metastases, stable disease, and a few long-term remissions have been seen with cancer vaccines.

## Recruiting the Immune System

Stimulating the body's immune system, also known as immunotherapy or biologic therapy, has been studied by cancer researchers for many years. Biologic agents like *interleukin-2* and *interferon alfa* have been approved by the FDA for use in cancer treatment, as have several monoclonal antibodies like Herceptin (trastuzumab) and Rituxan (rituximab). Continued research into better strategies for stimulating the immune system is underway. For example, clinical trials with monoclonal antibodies are continuing to see if these antibodies can be armed with radiation therapy, toxins, or chemotherapy agents to try to improve their effectiveness in cancer treatment. In these cases, the monoclonal antibodies can serve as a vehicle to get the therapy directly to the tumor cell. Some effectiveness has been proven with radioimmunotherapy.

Another area of immunotherapy research is with the use of *cytokines*, which are considered "immune system messengers." Research is being done on a cytokine called *granulocyte-monocyte colony stimulating factor (GM-CSF)*. GM-CSF is currently an FDA-approved drug used to boost the white blood cell count during a stem-cell or bone-marrow transplant. But it's now being studied in the treatment of melanoma to see if it can boost a type of immune cell, called an antigen-presenting cell, that supports the body's ability to cause an immune response.

A third new immunotherapy research strategy involves *adoptive immunotherapy*. This is a way genetically to instruct a human immune cell to seek and kill cancer cells. Cells called T-cells are taken from a patient and modified so that when they are returned to the patient, they'll recognize, target, and kill the patient's own tumor cells.

One interesting area of new research is the study of how tumor cells defy the body's immune system over time. Scientists have discovered that tumor cells can "recruit" healthy cells to help protect them from the immune system. They have discovered that fetuses in utero secrete an enzyme called IDO that disables the mother's immune system so that her immune system won't view the developing baby as a foreign substance and try to rid the body of it. Scientists are now injecting this enzyme into mice and are finding that it stimulates the immune system—which could be very helpful in finding better treatments for cancer. In a few years, this concept may be ready to try on humans. There's hope that this could be another step in unlocking the mysteries of the immune system.

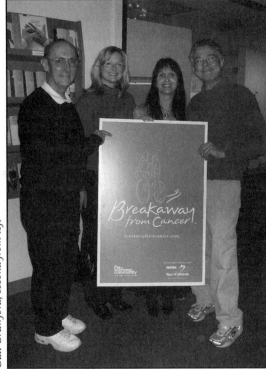

*Gail Crawford, second from left*

*I had genetic testing done and found out I do have the BRCA 2 gene. I elected to have an oopherectomy to prevent ovarian cancer. I also elected to have a second mastectomy with a tram-flap reconstruction to prevent additional breast cancer. I was told at diagnosis that I had a 15 percent chance to survive three years. I am now in my sixth year and have had no sign of active disease.*

*—GAIL CRAWFORD,*
*participant,*
*The Wellness Community -*
*Valley/Ventura*

## Targeting Genes

The common use of the term *gene therapy* relates to the application of genes to regulate cellular function or to correct cellular dysfunction. Another approach is to use the proteins expressed by certain genes as therapeutic agents to selectively kill cancer cells, while not harming healthy cells. Gene therapy in this way involves introducing or manipulating genetic material into a cell. It's an area of interest in cancer treatment research and is being studied through several approaches.

For example, missing or altered genes, like the p53 gene, which is considered a *tumor suppressor*, may be introduced into a cancer cell to suppress cancer cell growth. Or gene therapy may be used to try to stimulate the body's immune system or make cancer cells more sensitive to chemotherapy or radiation therapy, such as the way immunotherapy works. A third way that gene therapy is used for cancer treatment is with a "suicide gene" approach, where genes may be injected into cancer cells, and a drug is given later that activates cell death in the cancer cells that contain the injected genes. The "suicide genes" then cause the death of the cancer cell.

A common characteristic of gene therapy in cancer treatment is that genes must be transferred into cells by a "vehicle," or carrier, called a *vector*. Vectors are usually viruses that can be used safely to deliver the gene into the cancer cell. More research with gene therapy is underway to find the safest and most effective way to unleash this type of therapeutic advance.

Two new technologies are already being utilized in early clinical trials to determine their roles in the future of cancer treatment. These include *genomics*, which allows investigators to examine and identify the DNA of a cell, and *pharmacogenomics*, the study of inherited differences in how our bodies respond to different drugs. Anticipated benefits of pharmacogenomics include more powerful medicines, more accurate dosages, better vaccines, and better, safer drugs the first time.

## The Human Genome Project

In 1990, the Department of Energy and the National Institutes of Health started the U.S. *Human Genome Project* to identify genetic and environmental risk factors for all common diseases. This project was scheduled to last fifteen years, but effective resources and technological advances accelerated its completion date to 2003. The primary goals were to:

- Identify all 50,000–70,000 genes in human DNA
- Determine the sequences of 3 billion chemical base pairs that make up DNA
- Store this information in databases for further scientific testing

This research will eventually lead doctors and scientists to find better ways to prescribe treatments for each individual patient, based on his or her personal genetic make-up. Currently, targeted cancer therapies work only for a limited percent of the population. This research, as well as better diagnostic and genetic tests, will help improve the odds to treat more people accurately. There are still several barriers to using genetic testing and screening to better target cancer treatment at this time, including the protection of privacy and prevention of discrimination, as well as economics, because it's still very costly to use this type of personalized-treatment system.

### Linking Drug Response to Genetic Mutations

Some current research is showing the discovery of genetic mutations in some patients that may make those patients more responsive to certain targeted therapies. This may explain why with some therapies, a select subset of patients have a dramatic response, while other patients may not respond at all. This is one way of beginning to be able to "tailor" a cancer drug or regimen to a specific person. It is similar to the way Gleevec (imatinib mesylate) seems to work in certain leukemias and gastrointestinal stromal tumors that have specifically identified genetic mutations. As research continues, genetic testing may be used routinely to tell if a person is likely to respond to a certain drug or not.

## How Drug-Resistant Cancers Develop

Each new discovery in cancer can open doors of understanding for the future. It's long been known that cancers in some people can develop resistance to therapy, thereby making chemotherapy or, in some cases, novel therapies—like Gleevec—ineffective. When scientists discovered that some people with chronic myleogenous leukemia (CML) developed resistance to Gleevec, they gained new insight into how drug-resistant cancer mutations develop. A new compound, BMS-354825, has had some promising results in fighting chronic myeloid leukemia *after* Gleevec stops working. We continue to hope that new compounds such as this can be developed in order to side-step the drug-resistant mutations that cause other drugs to stop working.

## Proteomics

The study of the proteins found in cells, tissues, or organisms is called *proteomics* and is an evolving area for cancer researchers. Proteomics performs a similar task as genomics but examines cancer cell proteins instead of DNA. Proteins could serve as biomarkers that identify cancer cells and may be useful in detecting certain cancers. They may also help to predict how a cancer will respond to certain therapies and predict whether a cancer is likely to relapse.

For example, researchers have reported the ability to identify protein patterns in the blood of patients with ovarian cancer that may eventually lead to tests that detect ovarian cancer in early stages. Similar research is being conducted in prostate, breast, lung, and bladder cancer. Another recent study by the National Cancer Institute has reported the ability to use proteomics to identify patients who have *familial adenomatous polyposis*, which predisposes them to colon cancer. This identification process might tell doctors if the patient would be a good candidate for *chemoprevention* with the drug *celocoxib*. Scientists hope to determine whether proteomics can eventually lead to tailored cancer prevention for particular patients.

## Tissue Sample Research

Increasingly, people who have cancer are being asked if they would allow their blood samples and/or tumor tissue samples to be stored and studied. Many people are very willing to donate blood or tissue when they understand the important contributions these samples can provide to the future of cancer prevention, early detection, and treatment.

By studying the blood and tumor tissue at the cell's molecular level, scientists have been able to identify clues about how a tumor tissue grows, multiplies, and spreads. Scientists can study blood and tissue to look at the cell functions and signals, genetic factors, and proteins. This is allowing drugs to be developed that target these cell functions, signals, genes, and proteins in very specific ways.

Tissue sample research is a somewhat controversial area of discovery when it relates to the study of human *stem cells*, because of the ethical issues related to the means of obtaining some of the cells and tissue samples for research. Scientists, bioethicists, and politicians are debating these issues today with the hope of finding a common ground that benefits people with cancer and other serious diseases.

## Your Role in the Future of Cancer Research

People with cancer can play a valuable role in shaping the future of cancer care. By becoming knowledgeable about the latest treatment advances and by being willing to consider participation in clinical trials that are testing new therapies, you can contribute to improving cancer treatment. Even participation in studies involving the donation of blood or tissue samples, which often can be done with very little inconvenience to the patient, can make important contributions to the understanding of cancer prevention, early detection, and treatment.

### Stay Informed

Clinical developments and new discoveries in cancer happen frequently. For news and information on cancer diagnosis, treatment, and research, bookmark www.thewellnesscommunity. org and visit the site regularly.

### Patient Action Plan

- New therapies and treatments are being developed all the time
- Become your own "cancer researcher"—stay informed about new developments in cancer treatment
- Don't allow yourself to be overwhelmed by all of the new frontiers developing
- Consider becoming a tissue sample donor to contribute to the science of improving cancer treatment

*Chapter 7*

# Complementary and Alternative Medicine—Another Approach to Treatment

*Sure, the support groups are great, but for me, and to my amazement, these meditation and mind-body programs have changed my life. I feel like I'm on a path, and I honestly don't know where I'm going, but I'm comfortable with it. I feel less goal-oriented and more interested in learning. In addition, I want to move from victim to victor. Things will work out for me.... Maybe the cancer was needed for me to reflect on my life with the help of these programs.*

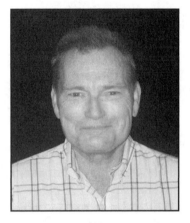

—JOHN STONE,
*participant, The Wellness Community - East Tennessee*

**m**OTIVATED BY THE DESIRE to improve their quality of life, get relief from symptoms and side effects, and feel more in control, many people with cancer are exploring complementary and alternative therapies in addition to mainstream cancer care. The National Center for Complementary and Alternative Medicine (NC-CAM), part of the National Institutes of Health, defines *Complementary and Alternative Medicines* (also known as *"CAM"*) as a "group of diverse medical and healthcare systems, practices, and products that are not presently considered to be part of conventional medicine." Some examples of CAM therapies include meditation, relaxation techniques, prayer, music and art therapy, acupuncture, biofeedback, and visualization.

CAM refers to more than specific treatments or practices. In essence, it's a broad social movement that continues to attract more people each year. A recent government survey showed that 36 percent of U.S. adults use some form of CAM. In a study done by Eisenberg et al. in 1998, it was estimated that 629 million visits were made to providers of CAM services in 1997, costing patients between $12–$20 billion in out-of-pocket expenses.

## Choices to Make

As a person with cancer or the caregiver for someone with cancer, you have many decisions to make about your treatment and lifestyle choices to increase the effectiveness of the treatments you're undergoing.

Some choices may be simple dietary changes and centering activities, such as prayer or yoga, while others may include vitamin or mineral supplements. Still, any choices you consider should be discussed with your doctor to make sure they won't interfere with any other treatments.

In addition to the choices you may discover in your own research, well-meaning friends and relatives may want to share information that they've found regarding a special alternative or complementary treatment for your kind of cancer. This chapter will help you navigate the various treatments available so that you and your doctor can make informed decisions about what's right for you.

## Alternative Medicines and CAM

Alternative medicines are different from CAM because they are used independently from conventional therapies. If someone opts to use herbal supplements to treat cancer, instead of chemotherapy or radiation, he or she would be using an alternative treatment. Alternative treatments may seem to offer hope when conventional treatments fail, but they're often unproven and can sometimes even be dangerous. If using an alternative treatment delays the use of a conventional treatment, then it can radically diminish the likelihood of remission and cure.

Some CAM therapies have been scientifically studied to see if they're effective, but many others haven't been studied, so it's still unknown whether they're safe or effective—or even how they work. As of now, no scientific studies have shown that complementary or alternative therapy alone can cure disease, but CAM can do the following:

- Relieve symptoms and side effects of cancer and its treatment
- Control pain and improve comfort
- Relieve stress and anxiety
- Enhance physical, emotional, and spiritual well-being
- Improve quality of life

As a complement to conventional treatments, CAM can be a useful tool. If you do choose to pursue CAM, make sure you learn as much as possible about your choice—and, as always, be sure to include your doctor and caregiver in your decision-making process.

| CAM CHOICE GUIDELINES |
| --- |
| Tell your doctor about your CAM use. |
| Carefully select the CAM practitioner to ensure quality and professionalism. |
| Know that products called "natural" are not necessarily safe. |
| Use information only from trusted resources. |
| Feel free to tell friends and family offering advice that you, your doctor, and your caregiver have come up with a game plan with which you are comfortable, but you appreciate their concern for you. |

There are five major categories of CAM: alternative medical systems, mind-body interventions, biologically based therapies, manipulative and body-based systems, and energy therapies. Let's explore each one in greater detail.

## Alternative Medical Systems: Achieving Mind-Body Harmony

Alternative medical systems include ayurveda, homeopathy, naturopathy, and traditional Chinese medicine. All of these are complete systems of theory and practice, and some have been used for centuries. A central theme to these systems is the goal of achieving harmony of mind and body. However, the basic assumptions and understandings of how disease unfolds in these systems don't jibe with current Western scientific understanding, which makes it more challenging to use these systems in conjunction with conventional medicine. However, you may still find elements in each system that are useful to you for CAM practices such as mind-centering, prayer, exercise, and relaxation.

## Ayurvedic Medicine

Ayurvedic medicine has been practiced primarily in the Indian subcontinent for 5,000 years. People are classified into one of three body types that determine which herbal remedies and dietary regimens they should use. A balanced consciousness is the key in ayurveda to prevent and treat disease. Yoga and meditation are techniques that are used to maintain and promote that balance.

## Homeopathic Medicine

Homeopathic medicine originated in Germany in the eighteenth century based on the principal that "like cures like." Small, highly diluted amounts of medicinal substances derived from plants, minerals, and animals are used to treat symptoms. In higher doses, these substances would actually cause symptoms. For instance, a poison ivy rash is treated by applying a solution of highly diluted poison ivy oil to the rash.

Clinical trials and systemic reviews have not found homeopathy to be a proven treatment for any medical condition. Some research indicates that homeopathy works due to the placebo effect: If the patient believes it will work, it may help him or her. But relying on this type of treatment on its own for any cancer could have negative consequences.

## Naturopathic Medicine

Naturopathic medicine includes many approaches to healing, including dietary modifications, massage, exercise, stress reduction, acupuncture, and conventional medicine. Practitioners believe that if a healthy internal environment exists, the body will heal itself.

Effectiveness of various methods varies, but many naturopathic remedies are used in other types of CAM. There's no scientific evidence that naturopathic medicine cures cancer or any other disease. Most methods within this practice won't harm you, but some herbal preparations can be toxic; for instance, fasting, limiting diet, and use of enemas could be dangerous if used excessively. Relying on naturopathic medicine as your sole treatment against cancer could also have negative consequences. However, massage, exercise, and stress reduction are all excellent for overall health, and when used in conjunction with treatment planned between you and your doctor, can be highly beneficial.

## Traditional Chinese Medicine

Traditional Chinese Medicine (TCM) views the body as an ecosystem that needs to stay in balance; opposing forces in the system can cause imbalance, disrupt the flow of energy, or Chi, and produce illness.

The goal of TCM is to maintain and promote balance within the system to restore positive energy flow. Herbal remedies, acupuncture, massage, and meditative physical exercise are all used as treatment. While the anti-cancer effects of TCM may be limited, many practices, such as acupuncture, have been shown to reduce side effects of cancer treatments, such as nausea and stress. Acupuncture has also been shown to be effective when combined with drugs for controlling postoperative pain in some patients.

More research is needed to assess the effectiveness of herbal remedies and other TCM practices.

## Mind-Body Interventions

Mind-body interventions are the second category in the five major types of CAM. Different techniques are used to influence the mind's ability to affect bodily function and systems. Mind-body interventions with which you may be familiar include prayer, meditation, guided imagery, and art, music, or dance therapy.

*Prayer* for health reasons is utilized by 43 percent of CAM users. The impact of prayer, spirituality, and religion on the well-being of cancer patients and their loved ones is an area of increasing study and interest.

*Meditation* relaxes the body and calms the mind, often creating a feeling of well-being. Different types of meditation include Zen, Vipassana, and Transcendental. Meditation can be self-directed or guided. It involves being in a quiet place and focusing on an object of meditation that may be breath, a mantra, or the physical sensations of slow walking.

*Guided imagery* practitioners help patients train the mind to produce a physiological or psychological effect using images and symbols.

Though there's no scientific evidence to prove that meditation treats cancer or any other disease, when used on a regular basis it's been shown to have some beneficial physiological and psychological effects. Clinical trials have found meditation useful in reducing anxiety, stress, blood pressure, chronic pain, and insomnia.

## Biologically Based Therapies

Biologically based therapies use substances that are found in nature, including herbs, certain foods or diets, and vitamins. Examples include dietary supplements, herbal products, and other "natural"—but unproven—therapies. Remember, a "natural" product does NOT *necessarily* mean a "safe" product! Please be aware that herbal products and vitamins may keep other medicines, such as chemotherapy, from doing what they are supposed to do. For example, research on St. John's wort, sometimes taken for depression, shows it may cause certain anticancer drugs NOT to work well.

*Dietary supplements* may include vitamins, minerals, herbs or other botanicals, amino acids, and substances such as *enzymes*, organ tissues, and *metabolites*. Dietary supplements come in many forms, including extracts, concentrates, tablets, capsules, gel caps, liquids, and powders. They're considered foods, not drugs, so there are no regulations controlling their safety, content, quality, or dose recommendations. The U.S. Food and Drug Administration (FDA) doesn't require manufacturers to print side effects on the labels of these products, or to remove them from the market, unless they're proven unsafe.

Dietary supplements have different active substances, so their effectiveness must be assessed individually. The American Cancer Society (www.cancer.org) has an extensive listing of dietary supplements on its Web site, and offers guidance through advice given by supporters and critics.

*Herbal products* are used in many different types of natural medicine. In the United States, herbal medicine generally refers to a system of medicine that uses European or North American plants. Ayurvedic medicine uses plants from India, and Traditional Chinese Medicine uses plants from China. Modern herbalists often use plants from many different regions of the world. Because herbs and roots have different active substances, their effectiveness must be evaluated individually.

## Manipulative and Body-Based Systems

Manipulative and body-based systems are practices based on physical manipulation and/or movement of one or more parts of the body. Examples include chiropractic or osteopathic manipulation and massage. There could be great risk associated with these types of therapies if a patient has bone metastases. As with any CAM treatments, you should consult with your physician first before utilizing these therapies.

*Chiropractic practices* focus on the relationship between bodily structure—primarily that of the spine—and function, and how that relationship affects health. Chiropractors use physical manipulation as an integral treatment tool. There's no scientific evidence that chiropractic treatment cures cancer or any other disease. However, it's been shown to help treat lower back pain and other pain due to muscle or bone problems—and it can promote relaxation and stress reduction. But complications can occur in a small number of cases.

*Osteopathic practice* is a form of conventional medicine emphasizing diseases that arise in the musculoskeletal system. It's grounded in a belief that the body's systems work together, and disturbances in one system can affect the functioning of another. Some osteopathic physicians practice a full-body system of hands-on manipulation to alleviate pain, restore function, and promote health and well-being. There is little scientific evidence that osteopathy is effective in treating cancer, or any other condition, except musculoskeletal problems. Some reports suggest that people with bone cancer should not use osteopathy.

*Massage* is when therapists manipulate and knead muscle and connective tissue to enhance function of those tissues, and promote relaxation and well-being. It can be used to relieve joint pain, reduce stiffness, rehabilitate injured muscles, and reduce pain. Recent studies suggest that massage can lower levels of stress, anxiety, depression, and pain. It may also have effects on fatigue, blood pressure, and quality of sleep. Massage that is conducted by a trained, licensed professional is regarded as safe. In the past, there was concern that people with cancer should not receive massage because tissue manipulation might cause cancer cells to migrate. No evidence has been found, however, to suggest that this will occur.

## Energy Therapies

*Energy therapies* are based on a theory that there are energy fields around the human body. It is believed that by changing the energy fields by manual manipulation, such as QiGong or healing touch, disease can be eliminated. Overall, energy therapies are considered to be questionable alternative therapies as far as treating disease, although many people with cancer relate that they find these practices to be helpful in reducing stress.

> There are two types of energy therapies:
> * *Biofield therapies* are meant to influence energy fields that theoretically surround and penetrate the body. Examples include QiGong, Reiki, and therapeutic touch
> * *Bioelectromagnetic-based therapies* involve using electromagnetic fields. Examples include pulsed fields, magnetic fields, or alternating current/direct current fields

*QiGong* is a component of Traditional Chinese Medicine that combines movement, meditation, and regulation of breathing to enhance the flow of Qi (an ancient term referring to "vital energy") in the body, improve blood circulation, and enhance immune function. There is no scientific evidence showing that QiGong is effective in treating cancer or any other disease; however, it may be useful to enhance quality of life. According to limited scientific literature, QiGong may reduce chronic pain for a short period of time and relieve anxiety.

*Reiki* is a Japanese word representing Universal Life Energy. Reiki is based on the belief that when spiritual energy is channeled through a reiki practitioner, the patient's spirit is healed, which in turn heals the physical body. No scientific studies show that reiki is effective for treating cancer or any other disease. However, it too may be useful as a complementary therapy to help reduce stress and improve quality of life.

Much like reiki, *therapeutic* or *healing touch* is derived from an ancient technique called "laying-on of hands," based on the premise that it is the healing force of the therapist that affects the patient's recovery. Healing is promoted when the body's energies are in balance, and, by passing their hands over the patient, healers can identify energy imbalances. There's no evidence to support that therapeutic touch (TT) balances or transfers energy, because very few well-designed studies of TT have been conducted. While one study published in the *Journal of the American Medical Association* (*JAMA*, 1998) demonstrated that experienced TT practitioners were unable to detect the energy fields of the investigator, TT is taught in many nursing schools and is still widely practiced. Some patients have found that it may help reduce anxiety and increase feelings of well-being. Many researchers believe that these results are due to the placebo effect, and that there's no consistent training or certifying organization to ensure the level of practice of the provider.

*Electromagnetic fields* (EMFs) are "invisible lines of force" that surround all electrical devices. Practitioners claim disease occurs when electromagnetic frequencies or fields of energy within the body are "out of balance." They believe electromagnetic imbalances disturb the body's chemistry. By applying electrical energy from outside the body, usually with electronic devices, practitioners say they can correct these imbalances. However, there's no scientific evidence that electromagnetic therapy is effective in diagnosing or treating cancer or any other disease; many of the alternative electronic devices promoted to cure disease have not been scientifically proven to be effective.

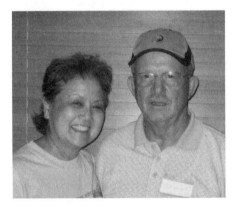

*I'm now attending yoga classes with Pat Collins, whose classes are very gentle and relaxing but are teaching me to stretch properly to regain my health. I'm also attending a T'ai chi class, which I hope will help me regain my balance and help the peripheral neuropathy in my hands and feet.*

—MASAKO HOLLOWELL,
*participant, The Wellness Community - Foothills*

## Eastern Exercises

*Yoga* is a form of exercise, usually anaerobic, that involves a sequence of postures and breathing activities. It can relieve some symptoms associated with cancer and other chronic diseases. A system of personal development from the Hindu tradition, it combines dietary guidelines, physical exercise, and meditation to create "prana," or vital energy. Research has found yoga to be beneficial to control bodily functions like blood pressure, heart rate, respiration, and metabolism. It can lead to improved physical fitness and lower levels of stress.

*T'ai chi* is an ancient Chinese martial art form. It's a mind-body system that uses movement, meditation, and breathing to improve health and well-being. Research has shown that T'ai chi is useful for improving posture, balance, muscle mass and tone, flexibility, stamina, and strength in older adults. T'ai chi is also an effective method for reducing stress.

## The Controversy over Alternative Diets

Diet and vitamin cancer "cures" have not been found to be scientifically effective as cancer treatments. Still, nutrition during and after cancer treatment is frequently a subject that concerns or interests people with cancer, as well as their loved ones.

It's hard to make sense of all the available information related to anticancer diets, though there are several popular approaches worthy of a closer look. Please remember that none of these approaches has been scientifically proven to prevent or eliminate cancer. Still, you might find that a registered dietician can be helpful in improving your nutritional practices during cancer treatment and beyond.

*Macrobiotic diet:* A vegetarian diet consisting predominantly of whole grains and cereals (50–60 percent), cooked vegetables and organic fruits (20–25 percent), and soups made with vegetables, seaweed, grains, beans, and miso (5–10 percent). Proponents believe that such a diet can prevent and cure disease, including cancer, and enhance feelings of well-being, though there have been no clinical trials to show that a macrobiotic diet can indeed prevent or cure cancer. Earlier forms of the diet, which involved restricting the diet to brown rice and water, were associated with severe nutritional deficiencies.

*Fasting:* Fasting entails not eating any foods and drinking only water or fruit juice for two to five days, or sometimes longer. Practitioners believe that fasting cleanses the body of toxins, but this belief is not supported by scientific research. The body cannot distinguish between fasting and starvation, and cancer studies suggest fasting may actually promote tumors.

*Gerson Therapy*: Involves using coffee enemas and a special diet with supplements to cleanse the body and stimulate metabolism. It's based on the theory that disease is caused by the accumulation of toxic substances. No well-designed scientific studies have supported the beliefs behind Gerson Therapy.

> *I was so happy I could do all of this and not have to worry about what it would cost. I learned about visualization and gained a powerful tool for helping myself fight my cancer. I learned where my tumor was located and what the cancer looked like so I could set 'bombs' off all day to help destroy my tumor. I felt empowered by doing this along with my radiation and chemo. To this day, I will set off 'bombs' to make sure I keep the tumor dead.*

> —JANET CAMPBELL,
> *participant, The Wellness Community - South Bay Cities*

## If You Use CAM, You Should Know That...

- **Some CAM therapies are safe, but others are not.**

  The fact that a product is called "natural" does not necessarily mean it is "safe." For example, the safety of dietary supplements and herbs depends on the ingredients in the product, where those ingredients are from, and whether they have been contaminated during manufacturing. Herbs and supplements can interact with other medications or prevent them from working. For this and other reasons, it is critical to talk to your doctor about CAM therapies. Your doctor can help you to understand the risks and benefits of a therapy. Be aware that each person reacts differently to treatments, and all medical therapies can have risks

- **It's important to be an informed consumer.**

  Learn as much as you can about therapies you are thinking of trying. Understanding the risks, potential benefits, and evidence of effectiveness for CAM therapies is vital to your safety. For many CAM therapies, few scientific studies of their effectiveness have been conducted. However, the National Center for Complementary and Alternative Medicine (NCCAM) is a good source for learning about existing studies *(see Appendix for more detailed resource information)*. You can also use the Internet to search PubMed, a database of medical literature, which has a listing of brief summaries of CAM studies, developed by NCCAM and the National Library of Medicine. In some cases, you may be able to click on a link to view or purchase the full articles. Another database, International Bibliographic Information on Dietary Supplements, is useful for finding scientific literature about dietary supplements

- **Information from Web sites should be viewed with a critical eye.**

  The Internet is a wonderful resource that allows you to obtain volumes of information with the click of a mouse, but not all information on the Internet is accurate. For this reason, it is important to evaluate Web sites with a critical eye. Look for sites that have been established by government agencies, universities, or reputable medical or health-related associations. Educational sites are more credible than those designed to sell a product. Information on the Web site should include clear references from scientific journals; personal stories are not adequate to back up statements. The information should also be current and recently updated. Be skeptical of sites that ask you for money or make claims that sound "too good to be true"

- **The federal government is a good resource for information about therapies you are considering.**

  If you are considering a therapy, check with the FDA's Web site, www.fda.gov, to see if it has information about that therapy. The FDA's Center for Food Safety and Applied Nutrition Web site has information about dietary supplements at www.cfsan.fda.gov. You can also visit the FDA's Web site on recalls and safety alerts at www.fda gov/opacom/7alerts.html. The Web site of the Federal Trade Commission (FTC), www.ftc.gov, offers information about consumer alerts for fraudulent therapies. Also, visit the NCCAM Web site, www.nccam.nih.gov, to see if it has information on the therapy

- **You can always check a CAM practitioner's credentials.**

  Licensed and credentialed practitioners can provide higher quality care than unlicensed ones. Credentials don't ensure that a practitioner is competent, but they show that he or she has met certain standards to treat patients.

  The training, skill, and experience of the practitioner

affect safety, so ask your physician or someone you believe is knowledgeable regarding CAM for recommendations.

Hospitals and medical schools sometimes keep lists of area CAM practitioners, and some may have a CAM center or CAM practitioners on staff. You may want to contact a professional organization for the type of practitioner you're seeking. Finally, many states have regulatory agencies or licensing boards that may be able to tell you about practitioners in your area

### Quackwatch and Other Watchdog Groups May Be Helpful

Quackwatch, Inc. is one example of a non-profit organization that aims to identify health-related frauds, myths, fads, and fallacies. This group primarily tries to expose quackery or "pretenders in medical skill, those who talk pretentiously without sound knowledge of the subject discussed." Quackwatch is useful for gaining background information on a questionable CAM topic or when information's difficult or impossible to find elsewhere. The services mentioned above may be found on www.quackwatch.org.

### Patient Action Plan

This helpful "to-do" list comes from the American Cancer Society's "Overview of Complementary and Alternative Therapies," found at www.cancer.org:

- Gather as much information as possible on your own. Seek information from reputable, credible sources on the potential benefits and risks of the treatment you are considering
- When you share this information with your doctor, do it in a non-confrontational manner
- Let him or her know that you are considering an alternative or complementary treatment and that you want to make sure it will not interfere with the treatment he or she has prescribed
- Develop a list of questions, and bring it, along with any literature you wish to discuss with your doctor. Ask your doctor to be a supportive partner in your education and treatment process
- Bring a friend or relative with you to the doctor's office

to be supportive of you. He or she can also help you communicate with your doctor and alleviate some of the stress of having to make decisions alone

- Listen to what your doctor has to say, and try to understand his or her perspective. If the treatment you are considering will cause problems with your conventional treatment, discuss safer alternatives together
- Don't delay or forgo conventional therapy. If you are considering stopping or not taking conventional treatment, please discuss this decision with your doctor. Remember that you may be giving up the only proven treatment
- Be sure to ask your doctor what conventional methods exist for treating the side effects or symptoms you are experiencing. Remember that many supportive medical treatments exist
- If you are taking dietary supplements, make a complete list of what dose you are taking of each supplement. Many supplements can interact in potentially harmful ways with conventional cancer treatment, so be sure to be conscientious about your supplement use. Report any changes to your healthcare team
- If you are pregnant or breastfeeding, ask about the risks and effects of complementary or alternative methods. Never give herbal medicines to children
- Ask your doctor to help you identify possible fraudulent products

## Chapter 8

# Clinical Trials

*I participated in a Phase III randomized double-blind trial of epidermal growth factor receptor antagonist ZD1839. I have now finished treatment [for lung cancer] and must go back every three months for a check. [Through it all], my experience at The Wellness Community has been educational—I've met many new friends and have attended wonderful special meetings and classes. It's one of the best things I have experienced since finding out about my lung cancer.*

—ROBERT FARQUHAR,
*participant, The Wellness Community - Greater Columbus*

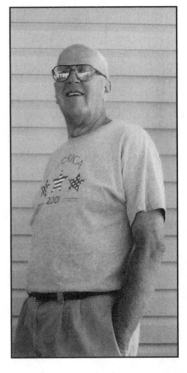

URING THE COURSE OF your treatment, your doctor may suggest that you consider being part of a clinical trial. This doesn't mean that you're being asked to be a human guinea pig, or that there aren't any other treatment options left. Rather, a clinical trial is usually considered when there is some reason to believe that the newer treatment currently under study might be a good option for you.

Before you consider giving your consent to participate in a clinical trial, you should learn as much as possible about what the treatments are, how they are developed, and what the risks and benefits are to each new treatment. Ask questions until you're sure you can make the best decision possible regarding your treatment possibilities.

## How New Cancer Treatments Are Developed and Tested

Before cancer treatments are available to the general public, research studies must show therapies are both safe and effective. The first step in this process occurs through basic research in the laboratory with preclinical testing in cell lines, tissues, and animal models of human cancer. Results from laboratory testing must demonstrate that the new intervention might work against cancer before studies are done in people. The next step involves human research studies, which are commonly referred to as *clinical trials*.

*People participating in clinical trials may be the first to benefit from a new treatment. The majority of studies in cancer are done in clinical trials conducted by the National Cancer Institute (NCI), cancer centers, and the pharmaceutical industry. But did you know that 85 percent of cancer patients aren't even aware that clinical trials may be a treatment option for them?*

## What Are Clinical Trials?

Clinical trials test promising new treatments, seek improvements to current treatments, or aim to detect or prevent cancer recurrence. Clinical trial participants make an important contribution to the future of cancer care.

Before a new treatment method for cancer is made available to the public, it must undergo a clinical trial, and any new treatment must successfully complete each of three phases of trials before the U.S. Food and Drug Administration (FDA) approves it for general use.

*Phase I* trials help researchers determine the best way to give a new treatment (by mouth, injection, or IV drip, for instance) and the most appropriate dosage. These trials also establish whether a treatment has any potentially harmful side effects. Only a few people participate in this stage.

*Phase II* trials evaluate whether the new treatment actually has a positive effect against a particular type of cancer. In general, if at least 20 percent of participants respond well to the treatment, the new therapy undergoes further evaluation.

*Phase III* trials compare the new treatment to the best existing treatment for a particular type of cancer. If eligible, many people—from the hundreds to even the thousands—can participate. Phase III trials can involve, for example, adding a new drug to an already-proven combination of drugs to see if the combination is more effective. It's important to know that every participant in a Phase III trial receives either the current standard treatment *or* the new treatment. People who are eligible for a clinical trial and choose to participate are informed of the possible risks and benefits and are protected through laws that guarantee a participant's right to leave the trial at any time.

### Research Goals in Clinical Trials
*Phase I*: Is the drug safe?
*Phase II*: Does the drug work?
*Phase III*: How does the drug compare to the best standard of care?

### Types of Clinical Trials
*Prevention trials* test new approaches, such as medications, vitamins, or other supplements, that doctors believe may lower the risk of developing a certain type of cancer. Most prevention trials are conducted with healthy people who haven't had cancer. Some trials are conducted with people who have had cancer and want to prevent recurrence (return of cancer), or reduce the chance of developing a new type of cancer.

*Screening trials* study ways to detect cancer earlier. They are often conducted to determine whether finding cancer before it causes symptoms decreases the chance of dying from the disease. These trials involve people who do not have any symptoms of cancer.

*Diagnostic trials* study tests or procedures that could be used to identify cancer more accurately, and they usually include people who have signs or symptoms of cancer.

*Treatment trials* are conducted with people who have cancer. They are designed to answer specific questions about, and evaluate the effectiveness of, a new treatment or a new way of using a standard treatment. These trials test many types of treatments, such as new drugs, vaccines, new approaches to surgery or radiation therapy, or new combinations of treatments.

*Quality-of-life* (also called supportive care) *trials* explore ways to improve the comfort and quality of life of cancer patients and cancer survivors. These trials may study ways to help people who are experiencing nausea, vomiting, sleep disorders, depression, or other effects from cancer or its treatment.

*Genetic studies* are sometimes part of another cancer clinical trial. The genetics component of the trial may focus on how genetic makeup can affect detection, diagnosis, or response to cancer treatment.

*Population- and family based genetic research studies* differ from traditional cancer clinical trials. In these studies, researchers look at tissue or blood samples, generally from families or large groups of people, to find genetic changes that are associated with cancer. People who participate in genetics studies may or may not have cancer, depending on the study. The goal of these studies is to help understand the role of genes in the development of cancer.

*Source: National Cancer Institute*

## How Does a Drug Gain FDA Approval?

If the data obtained from a completed Phase III trial shows a new treatment to be safe and effective, the sponsor of the trial can then submit an application to the FDA for approval of the treatment. Scientists at the FDA analyze the data brought to them to ensure that safety and efficacy have been established. After extensive review, if the FDA is satisfied with the results, approval is granted and the drug then becomes available on the market.

**Find a Clinical Trial**

The Wellness Community is proud to provide a free and confidential clinical trials search engine that offers information about clinical trials currently available throughout the U.S. To find a clinical trial, visit www.thewellnesscommunity.org/clinical.trials/clinical.trial.asp, or call 1-800-814-8927.

## Expanded-Access Programs

For a very small percentage of treatments in clinical trials, the FDA has recently begun to offer *"expanded-access"* programs. These programs make investigational therapies available—outside of the traditional clinical trial setting—to people with serious or life-threatening illnesses and without other treatment options, even before these drugs are formally approved by the FDA for the public's use.

Expanded-access programs for new treatments make new, promising therapies available to more patients, but these programs are also designed under regulatory supervision to maintain data collection on important drug safety and efficacy information, and they are only offered when the FDA feels that expanded access won't compromise a patient's safety or the integrity of the clinical-trial evaluation.

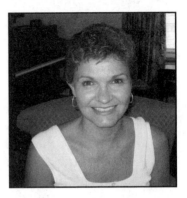

*I was the last person chosen for [a] Phase I/II trial of PR1 peptide vaccine. The support I received [at TWC] helped me to grow spiritually throughout that ordeal. I now go to my local oncologist monthly for CBCs. If my counts are good, I run out the door for another month. There are no promises, projections, or probabilities offered for the duration of my remission. The drug I received is too new for that. I'm learning to live one day at a time.... I try to make the best of that, make reasonable plans for the future, and then turn it over to God.*

—KIMBERLY HENRY,
*The Wellness Community - East Tennessee*

## About Informed Consent

Before you join a clinical trial, a healthcare professional will explain the purpose of the trial and what you'll be asked to do. You can ask questions about the trial and will be given a consent form to read and sign. The informed consent process begins with the initial explanation from your doctor, the document you sign to start treatment, and then ongoing information provided to you throughout the course of your treatment.

The consent form must include the following information:

- A statement that the study involves research, an explanation of the purposes of the research, the expected timeframe of participation, a description of the procedures, and identification of procedures that are experimental
- Facts about how the clinical trial is done

- Any likely risks to you from the treatment
- A description of any benefits to you or others that may reasonably be expected from the research
- A statement describing the extent, if any, to which confidentiality of your records will be kept
- An explanation of alternative options, if any exist
- Any likely side effects from the treatment
- For trials involving more than minimal risk: an explanation of potential injuries, compensation—if any—available due to injury, treatments available if injury occurs, and resources for further information
- An explanation of whom to contact for answers to questions about the research and participants' rights and about research-related injury to the participant
- A statement that participation is voluntary, refusal to participate will not have penalties or loss of benefits to which you would otherwise be entitled, and you may discontinue participation at any time without penalty or loss of benefits to which you would be otherwise entitled

Here are some important questions you should ask your doctor before choosing to participate in a clinical trial:

- What's the purpose of the study?
- Why would it be important to me?
- What kinds of tests and treatments are done as part of the study?
- What are my potential benefits and risks compared to other treatment options?
- What are the eligibility requirements?
- How could the clinical trial affect my daily life?
- What will happen to my cancer with or without this new treatment?
- What are other treatment choices?
- How long will the study last?
- Will my insurance company, Medicare, Medicaid, or managed care plan cover the costs?
- Who will help me answer coverage questions?
- Will I have extra out-of-pocket costs due to the clinical trial?
- What type of long-term care and follow-up are part of the study?

**Benefits and Risks to Participation**

According to the National Cancer Institute, the benefits of participating in a clinical trial include the following:

- Participants have access to promising new approaches that often aren't available outside the clinical-trial setting
- The approach being studied may be more effective than the standard approach
- Participants receive regular and careful medical attention from a research team that includes doctors and other health professionals
- Participants may be the first to benefit from the new method under study
- Results from the study may help others in the future

The possible risks of participating in a clinical trial include the following:

- New drugs or procedures under study are not always better than the standard care to which they are being compared
- New treatments may have side effects or risks that doctors don't expect, or that are worse than those resulting from standard care
- Participants in randomized trials won't be able to choose the approach they receive
- Health insurance and managed care providers may not cover all patient care costs in a study
- Participants may be required to make more visits to the doctor than they would if they were not in the clinical trial

*Source: National Cancer Institute*

## Are You Protected During a Clinical Trial?

Research with humans is conducted according to strict scientific and ethical principles. Every clinical trial has a protocol or action plan that serves as a "recipe" for conducting the trial. The plan describes what will be done in the study, how it will be conducted, and why each part of the study is necessary. The same protocol is used by every doctor or research center taking part in the trial.

All clinical trials that are federally funded or that evaluate a new drug or medical device subject to FDA regulation must be reviewed and approved by an Institutional Review Board (IRB). Many institutions require that all clinical trials, regardless of funding, be reviewed and approved by a local IRB. The Board, which includes doctors, researchers, community leaders, and other members of the community, reviews the protocol to make sure the study is conducted fairly and participants aren't likely to be harmed. The IRB also decides how often to review the trial once it has begun. Based on this information, the IRB decides whether the clinical trial should continue as initially planned and, if not, what changes should be made. An IRB can stop a clinical trial if the researcher isn't following the protocol or if the trial appears to be causing unexpected harm to the participants. In order to make it widely available, an IRB can also stop a clinical trial if there's clear evidence that the new intervention is effective.

National Institutes of Health-supported clinical trials require data and safety monitoring. Some clinical trials, especially Phase III clinical trials, use a Data and Safety Monitoring Board (DSMB). A DSMB is an independent committee made up of statisticians, physicians, and patient advocates. The DSMB ensures that the risks of participation are as small as possible, makes sure the data is complete, and stops a trial if safety concerns arise or when the trial's objectives have been met.

## Who Pays for Clinical Trials?

*Source: National Cancer Institute*

Health insurance and managed care providers often do not cover the patient care costs associated with a clinical trial. What they cover varies by health plan and by study. Some health plans do not cover clinical trials if they consider the approach being studied "experimental" or "investigational." However, if enough data shows that the approach is safe and effective, a health plan may consider the approach "established" and cover some or all of the costs. Participants may have difficulty obtaining coverage for costs associated with prevention and screening clinical trials; health plans are currently less likely to have review processes in place for these studies. It may, therefore, be more difficult to get coverage for the costs associated with them. In many cases, it helps to have someone from the research team talk about coverage with representatives of the health plan.

Health plans may specify other criteria a trial must meet to be covered. The trial might have to be sponsored by a specified organization, be judged "medically necessary" by the health plan, not be significantly more expensive than treatments the health plan considers standard, or focus on types of cancer for which no standard treatments are available. In addition, the facility and medical staff might have to meet the plan's qualifications for conducting certain procedures, such as *bone marrow transplants*. More information about insurance coverage can be found on the NCI's *Clinical Trials and Insurance Coverage: A Resource Guide* Web page at www.cancer.gov/clinicaltrials/learning/insurance-coverage.

Many states have passed legislation or developed policies requiring health plans to cover the costs of certain clinical trials. For more information, visit the NCI's Web site at www.cancer.gov/clinicaltrials/developments/laws-about-clinical-trial-costs.

Federal programs that help pay the costs of care in a clinical trial include those listed below:

- Medicare reimburses patient care costs for its beneficiaries who participate in clinical trials designed to diagnose or treat cancer. Information about Medicare coverage of clinical trials is available at www.medicare.gov, or by calling Medicare's toll-free number for beneficiaries at 1–800–633–4227 (1–800–MEDICARE). The toll-free number for the hearing impaired is 1–877–486–2048. Also, the NCI fact sheet, *More Choices in Cancer Care: Information for Beneficiaries on Medicare Coverage of Cancer Clinical Trials*, is available at www.cancer.gov/cancertopics/factsheet/support/medicare

- Beneficiaries of TRICARE, the Department of Defense's health program, can be reimbursed for the medical costs of participation in NCI-sponsored Phase II and Phase III cancer prevention (including screening and early detection) and treatment trials. Additional information is available in the NCI fact sheet, *TRICARE Beneficiaries Can Enter Clinical Trials for Cancer Prevention and Treatment Through a Department of Defense and National Cancer Institute Agreement*. This fact sheet can be found at www.cancer.gov/cancertopics/factsheet/NCI/TRICARE

- The Department of Veterans Affairs (VA) allows eligible veterans to participate in NCI-sponsored prevention, diagnosis, and treatment studies nationwide. All phases and types of NCI-sponsored trials are included. The NCI fact sheet, *The NCI/VA Agreement on Clinical Trials: Questions and Answers*, has more information. It's available at www.cancer.gov/cancertopics/factsheet/NCI/VA-clinical-trials

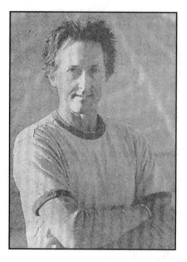

*With the help of The Wellness Community, I was able to muster the strength to 'dig deep' one more time, and in February 2004, I was to have an autologous stem-cell transplant at City of Hope National Medical Center. The transplant was a challenge and marked a turning point for me. It really became what amounted to a resurrection. The recovery process from this was a tough time, but a valuable one. I was lucky enough to be in the research protocol for this brand-new kind of transplant.... It has been described by the staff at City of Hope as an 'eleventh-hour save'—and it certainly felt like one to me.*

—Douglas Wilkey, Jr.,
*cancer survivor and participant,*
*The Wellness Community - Central Arizona*

## Research's Long-Term Impact on Patients

Information gathered from research studies in humans tells doctors which treatments, including dosages, schedules, and combinations, work and don't work in patients. Results from testing in clinical trials continue to determine the *standard of care*, a term for the treatment approach considered best in patients by the cancer community, according to their type and stage of cancer. Standard treatments typically have been studied in clinical trials that demonstrated a proven benefit to patients through an increase in survival, decrease in the size of the tumor or extensiveness of the disease, or improved quality of life through a reduction in side effects.

As we've said, many types of cancer are being treated as more of a chronic disease to be controlled over time. Even those cancers diagnosed in later stages are sometimes seen as serious life-threatening illnesses to be managed over the course of several years. Therefore, oncologists and patients are shifting their treatment strategies with the consideration of long-term health issues. This shift is directed toward the goal of enabling a person with cancer to function at his or her maximum level for as long as possible.

Treatment plans may be sequenced over a span of many years to prolong survival, and they include an assessment of how treatment side effects will be tolerated over time. Researchers will continue to study new treatments until every type of cancer can be prevented or cured.

**Patient Action Plan**
- **Partner with your physician.**
  Before deciding to enroll in a clinical trial, schedule a meeting to talk with your oncologist. Bring a family member or friend to help you address your questions and concerns
- **Find support.**
  Talk with others who have experience with a clinical trial. Your healthcare team or organizations such as The Wellness Community will help connect you with others who can share their experiences
- **Educate yourself.**
  There are organizations that provide up-to-date information about what's being studied and whether a cancer clinical trial is right for you. (*See Appendix for some helpful Web sites with information about specific trials*)

## Chapter 9

# Managing Symptoms and Side Effects

*A friend gave me a pink pig called 'Matilda.' For each treatment, I added an item to her. First was earrings, second was a rhinestone belly button. I continued [doing this] through eight treatments. My chemo nurse couldn't wait until my next treatment to see what I put on Matilda next.*

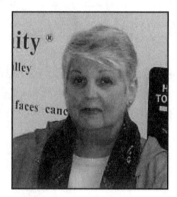

—Sally B. Frank,
*participant, The Wellness Community - Greater Lehigh Valley*

e VERY PERSON'S EXPERIENCE WITH cancer treatment is unique. You may not experience every possible side effect, but being aware of what *might* happen can help reassure you that certain side effects are "normal," and as a result, better prepare you for dealing with them.

More importantly, being better informed may enable you and your doctor to prevent or proactively manage side effects so they won't disrupt your treatment, decrease your quality of life, or even impact your possibility of recovery.

## "Is It the Cancer...or Something Else?"

People who've been diagnosed with cancer have learned rapidly that life, as they knew it, changed when they heard the words, "You've got cancer." Many patients have shared that, ever since their diagnosis, they've become very conscious of their bodies and the messages their bodies send to them. Some worry that maybe they stress too much about "every ache and pain." But how can you tell when something is wrong? Do you often wonder that an ache or other symptom might be a sign the cancer is progressing? It's important that you learn to read your physical signs, keep track of symptoms and side effects, and communicate with your healthcare team on a regular basis.

No question is ever too dumb to ask. More often than not, the signs and symptoms you're experiencing are temporary and related to the treatment you are receiving, as well as to the changes that are occurring in your body as it works to control or destroy the cancer.

If you experience a side effect from therapy, it doesn't mean that something is wrong or that the drugs you're taking aren't destroying the cancer cells. Nor does it mean that the cancer has necessarily progressed. However, it does mean that you must be vigilant and maintain open communication with your team so that you can be as proactive as possible in keeping your treatment on track—and committed to feeling as good as possible.

*The most important thing you can do is be a proactive participant in your own disease management.*

So often, we let our minds tell us something is worse than it really is. It's normal for you to fear that the cancer is growing or not going away. You may be feeling betrayed by your body becoming ill in the first place and have difficulty feeling you can ever trust it again. The good news is that there are some simple ways you can reclaim control over your reactions to these difficult stressors.

The easiest way to understand what you're experiencing is to be well informed. The Wellness Community's approach is an excellent way to learn to properly identify your symptoms and effectively communicate about their frequency, intensity, and extent to your physician. By knowing what potential side effects might happen, you can alert your doctor or nurse of their occurrence before they become severe and before you get yourself in a quandary over whether these concerns are related to the treatment or to the cancer itself.

Remember, this is where being Patient Active becomes so important. Be proactive in asserting what you need to prevent or control side effects. Be clear with your healthcare team about how any particular symptoms you are having may be impacting your day-to-day life. And don't forget, no one ever said that just because you have cancer you have to suffer; thanks to phenomenal advances in supportive treatments, cancer therapy doesn't have to be as miserable as you might think. You can do it! Be informed—take action!

## Staying on Schedule

It's important that your treatment remains on schedule. After all, you want to get through your treatment as quickly and successfully as possible, right? Having to postpone your treatment due to a low white blood cell count or other distressing side effects can leave you feeling disappointed, anxious, and fearful. Not only will managing side effects improve the way you feel during treatment, it could also make a difference in the outcome of your treatment.

In a recent study of 500 chemotherapy patients, 37 percent of those who experienced a delay due to a low white cell count said they found the delay to be "extremely" or "somewhat" stressful. Delays can be emotionally troubling for patients who become concerned that their cancer may progress while waiting to restart treatment. Thirty-one percent of patients surveyed who experienced a delay said they felt emotionally troubled enough to want to quit their treatment at some point (Mock et al.).

In addition to the emotional distress, changing or interrupting the delivery of a planned dose can impact a patient's physical well-being. Current research suggests that both dose timing and intensity can affect outcomes for some cancer patients. Giving lower doses, or giving doses over a longer period of time than initially planned, may even reduce the effectiveness of the treatment in some types of cancer.

*Fatigue has been a problem. . . . I have a daily schedule to get me out of bed before lunchtime, excluding the week following chemo. I attend my support group early on Mondays. Tuesdays, there's bridge and lunch. Wednesdays and Fridays, there are exercise classes for 'Building Bones.' In between times, I swim, read, walk the dogs, visit with friends, attend seminars on*

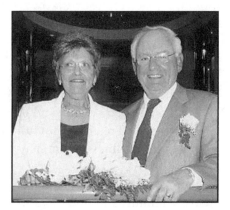

*current events, and do things of less interest such as laundry, shopping, and cleaning. I do keep busy.*

—STEFANIE MARKS,
*participant, The Wellness Community - Greater St. Louis*

## Fatigue

Nearly all people who are treated for cancer experience cancer-related fatigue. It is the most commonly registered complaint of patients with cancer and, frequently, the most distressing.

The National Comprehensive Cancer Network (NCCN) defines fatigue as "a distressing, persistent sense of tiredness or exhaustion that is not related to recent activity and interferes with the normal activities of daily living." The NCCN Guidelines recommend that you be assessed for the effects of fatigue at each visit with your doctor and as needed.

### How Much Fatigue Will I Experience—and for How Long?

It's difficult to predict how fatigued you will feel, because it tends to be different from person to person. Fatigue may be associated with treatment or may depend on when treatment is given. In most cases, you'll gradually begin to feel less fatigued when your treatment ends. Some therapies cause more fatigue than others, such as bone marrow or stem cell transplants, some biotherapies, and certain radiotherapies.

### What Can I Do to Avoid the Effects of Fatigue?

Part of managing fatigue is discovering the causes and putting a plan of action into place to deal with the fatigue during treatment. Your health-care team will want to know:

- If you're having problems with pain or difficulty sleeping
- Whether you're experiencing emotional distress or depression
- What your activity levels have been
- How well you're eating and drinking
- Whether you're anemic or at risk for anemia (low red blood cells)
- What other illnesses you may have or medications you're taking

It's important to be very honest about what medications (prescribed, herbals, vitamins, and other over-the-counter medicines) you're taking. Some medicines and combinations of medications can contribute to fatigue, and it's possible to adjust medicine regimens to avoid making the fatigue worse.

Experiencing the problem of fatigue is an undesirable but expected consequence of cancer treatment. Feeling fatigued isn't itself an indication that your cancer is worse. Discuss your problems of fatigue regularly with your healthcare team so that strategies can be put in place to help you.

> **Conserve Your Energy!**
> - Delegate tasks to others
> - Nap in the early afternoon—short power-naps, not long enough to interfere with nighttime sleep
> - Avoid caffeine in the evening
> - Schedule activities, or structure your routine to accomplish tasks
> - Keep a regular daily routine that is reasonable, considering your abilities
> - Take short walks, or do light exercise, if possible
> - Set realistic goals that you can meet without too much effort
> - Drink water during the day
> - Eat a well-balanced diet with frequent, small meals
> - Learn mind-body techniques to de-stress and relax
>
> Engage your family and friends in helping you accomplish tasks that are important to you, and permit others to relieve you of responsibilities and work that can be completed for you. You should view this as a good opportunity to take control of your life and the situation.

## What about Exercise?

There is a large body of research demonstrating the benefits of exercise on the emotional and physical side effects of cancer and its treatment. Exercise reduces fatigue, distress, and depression; it also helps with weight control, endurance, and your ability to do the things that are meaningful and important to you.

While many healthcare practitioners may encourage you to exercise, they may not know exactly what to tell you to do. You can be Patient Active and ask your physician for a referral to a physical therapist or cancer rehabilitation program. If you don't ask, these extended services may not be readily offered.

Walking is one safe, easy way to stay strong and get healthier during cancer treatment. Because cancer treatments may make you feel fatigued, exercise can help you generate more energy and feel physically and emotionally equipped to deal with your illness and life. While exercise won't make your cancer go away, it's something you can do for yourself to feel better, get through treatment more easily, and stay healthy after your treatment ends.

Some cancer treatments and their side effects might make it difficult for you to exercise. For example, if you have anemia that's not corrected with medication (red blood cell growth factors), you may experience shortness of breath. If you walk more slowly and take rest breaks, you can still receive the benefits of exercise. It's also okay if you start with simply walking across the room a few times a day. You'll get stronger if you're dedicated to being an active cancer survivor.

## How Do I Start to Exercise?

Start slowly, and be patient. Exercise during cancer treatment is a balance, and more isn't always better. Start your exercise routine well below what you believe you can do, and progress in step-by-step fashion. In time, you'll be able to do more of the things you want to do with less effort.

Long after treatment is behind you, it's important to be proactive in maintaining your health. Exercise can help you maintain a healthy body weight and reduce your risks for heart disease and diabetes—and perhaps even the risk of a cancer recurrence. It's always one of the most important things you can do for yourself!

## Hair Loss, or Alopecia

Hair loss, also known as *alopecia*, has long been an indicator that a person has cancer. Experiencing hair loss is a deeply personal and upsetting experience for most people. It's normal to be distressed about the loss of your hair and how it affects your appearance. Discussing your concerns with your healthcare team and finding ways to manage the loss is important for you to do.

Not all treatment for cancer will cause hair loss—and most hair loss isn't permanent. You should ask if your treatment causes hair loss so that you can prepare for it, if it's an expected side effect. Hair loss usually begins ten to fourteen days following the first treatment; it's difficult to predict exactly how it will happen, but it may gradually thin or fall out in large clumps. You're also likely to lose hair all over your body at the same time. In most cases, your hair will grow back when your treatment has been completed. Many times, the texture and color of your new hair will be slightly different.

## How Can I Manage Hair Loss?

If you plan to get a wig, visiting your hairdresser or wig store before you lose your hair is a good idea. That way, you can best match your natural hair to the wig. However, you may also choose a wig that is completely different from your real hair.

Some insurance companies will supplement the cost of a wig, but you must submit a prescription written by your physician for a *cranial* or *hair prosthesis*. Frequently, cancer treatment centers will have "wig banks" where you can get a rehabilitated or new wig for free, or at low cost.

Alternatives to wigs include hats, scarves, and turbans. You should get into the habit of protecting your head from the sun by applying sunscreen and wearing a covering of some kind over your head. It's also important to protect yourself from loss of body heat when the weather is cool by wearing a hat or other head covering.

Many people will choose to get a very short haircut or to shave their heads before they begin to lose their hair. In doing this, you'll have the opportunity to control how the hair loss will occur and have time to see the "new look" before anyone else.

> *For those of you who are losing your hair, my suggestion is to SHAVE YOUR HEAD! I am bald right now for the second time. I wear a lot of baseball caps because they're easy and comfortable. I lost my hair for six weeks the first time, due to chemo. I cut my hair short, but it still fell out in gobs, got under my clothes, and made my skin itch. Would you believe I was wearing a shower cap while making dinner? Fear of my hair falling into the food…how gross is that? Shaving my head actually made my life better. I have less stress and anxiety—and it's more comfortable! Our older dog finds my bald head rather amusing. She now loves to lick the top of my head! However, she's now prone to wanting to lick ALL people with bald heads. We're lucky to have friends with a sense of humor!*
>
> —Diane Gresham,
> *participant, The Wellness Community - Greater Boston*

## Can I Prevent Hair Loss?

You can't prevent hair loss, but you can take some precautions to prevent damage to the hair that remains, such as avoiding permanents or coloring, curlers, and hairdryers on high heat settings. You should use a mild shampoo, soft hairbrushes, and mild lotions. The use of ice or other methods to prevent hair loss should be avoided. Any products suggested to you should be discussed with your doctor prior to use to avoid any possible harm.

## Infections and Fever

Infections can be one of the most serious side effects of treatment, and it should be your goal to avoid them whenever possible. They can lead to hospitalization, which can be costly and disruptive, keeping you from your daily activities and loved ones. At their most serious, infections can be life-threatening.

Fever that occurs when your blood counts are low is considered a cancer care emergency, requiring prompt medical attention—so call your doctor immediately if this occurs.

A fever is the body's natural response against invaders (such as viruses, bacteria, and fungi) that cause infection, and it can be the first sign of infection. Infection can occur because the drugs that fight cancer cells may also cause a decrease in the normal white blood cells, called neutrophils, in the blood. Radiation to your spine, hips, or pelvis could also cause a decrease in white blood cells. The condition when your white blood count is really low is called *neutropenia.*

Throughout your cancer treatment, your blood will be drawn and tested frequently. While your medical team is keeping track of your white blood, platelet, and red blood cell count, it's important for you to keep track, as well. Try keeping track of your complete blood count (CBC) on a CBC Log, such as the one included in the Appendix of this book, to assist you in monitoring this critical aspect of your care.

While white blood cells fight infection, red blood cells transport oxygen throughout your blood stream and clot your blood with *platelets* when you bleed. If the number of white cells in your blood drops, you could develop a serious infection and end up in the hospital. An infection might also mean a disruption in your treatment schedule or a reduction in a vital dose of chemotherapy.

## Symptoms of Infection

A fever—the body's natural response against invaders such as viruses, bacteria, and fungus—is often one of the first symptoms of infection. Fever that occurs when your white blood cell count is too low is considered an emergency, requiring prompt medical attention. When you're on chemotherapy, take your temperature daily. If you have a fever higher than 100.4°F (38°C), call your doctor or nurse immediately, because it could mean that you have an infection.

Also report these symptoms of infection to your doctor or nurse right away:

- Chills, shaking, sweating
- Cough, sore throat, shortness of breath, and/or chest pain
- Redness, warm skin, pain or swelling around a wound or catheter site (PICC line, Port-a-cath, or other central line)
- Loose bowels or diarrhea for more than twenty-four hours
- Pain or a burning sensation during urination or pain in the back above the waist
- Unusual vaginal discharge or itching
- Mouth ulcers

You'd be considered in a high-risk category for neutropenia if: you're on chemotherapy known to decrease the number of white blood cells; you already have a low white blood cell count or previously received chemotherapy or radiation; you are age sixty-five or older; or you have another condition that affects your immune system (Fortner et al.).

One of the most effective ways to monitor signs of infection is to take your temperature every day—ideally around the same time during your treatment cycle. Ask your doctor what time of day is best. *If your temperature is over 100.4°F (38°C), call your doctor or nurse immediately to determine whether you have an infection.* The sooner you detect an infection, the more likely you'll minimize disruption to your treatment schedule. Use the Temperature Log provided in the Appendix to track your temperature on a daily basis.

You'll be susceptible to infection as long as you have a reduced number of white blood cells circulating in your blood stream. The period of time it takes for white blood cells to recover varies, depending on the type and dose of chemotherapy, as well as on your body's own ability to replace the damaged cells.

## Preventing Infection

The most important way to avoid the spread of infection-causing bacteria is to wash your hands frequently. Take time to scrub your hands thoroughly with soap and warm water—it's the friction that kills bacteria. Your doctor may prescribe a white blood cell growth factor medication to help you produce more white blood cells and reduce the period of time you're at risk. These medications are given after every cycle of chemotherapy to stimulate the bone marrow to produce more white blood cells. White blood cell growth factors can ease achiness and some flu-like symptoms. They can also help you get your treatment as planned and at the full dose, ultimately improving your chances for a cure.

## What's the Treatment for Infection?

If you develop an infection, most likely you will be treated with antibiotics. In some cases, hospitalization may be necessary. Obviously, you want to spend as little time in the hospital as possible. Working and/or managing other roles and responsibilities throughout treatment make it even more vital to be vigilant about preventing infection.

## Taking Steps to Avoid Infection

Fortunately, you may be able to prevent a dangerous infection before it occurs. If your white blood cell count remains too low, your oncologist may need to reduce or delay your next treatment. Your doctor may also prescribe medication to help you produce more white blood cells from the very beginning, reducing the period of time that you might be at risk of infection.

Many patients take a medication that stimulates the growth of white blood cells, such as *Filgrastim*, from the start of chemotherapy until their white count recovers. Be sure to ask your doctor if this type of medication would be helpful in your treatment regimen.

Like any medication, a white blood cell stimulator is only effective when you take the right dosage for the right number of days. Your doctor will determine the appropriate dosage based upon your body weight. You can expect to begin taking a white blood cell growth factor twenty-four hours after your last chemotherapy treatment of your current cycle. You would then continue taking it for up to ten days. Again, be sure to ask your doctor if this type of medication would be helpful in your treatment regimen.

Once your doctor prescribes a medication to prevent low white cell counts, it's important to continue receiving it following every chemotherapy cycle. Research has shown that people who experience neutropenia after a chemotherapy treatment are more likely to experience neutropenia again with future chemotherapy treatments.

**Other Preventive Actions:**
- Avoid low white blood cell counts in advance
- Wash your hands often during the day
- Clean your rectal area gently but thoroughly after each bowel movement
- Avoid crowds and individuals who may have diseases you can catch, such as colds, chicken pox, and the flu
- Avoid cutting your skin: use an electric shaver instead of a razor, don't tear or cut the cuticles of your nails, and be careful when handling knives
- Use oil or lotion to soften your skin if it becomes dry and cracked
- Clean cuts and bruises with warm water and an antiseptic

**Did You Know That:**
- Too much rest, as well as too little rest, contributes to increased feelings of fatigue?
- Too little activity, as well as too much activity, can cause feelings of fatigue?
- Everyday energy expenditure in activity is the most potent known regulator of the body's energy systems? (With energy, it's a "use it or lose it" proposition)
- Feeling fatigued can make you feel more distressed about other symptoms or concerns?
- How you feel about other symptoms or concerns can lead to feelings of fatigue?

## Anemia

Anemia occurs when your red blood cell count is lower than normal. *Hemoglobin (Hgb)* is an important part of your red blood cells. At normal levels, hemoglobin supplies your body with the oxygen it needs to work properly. When hemoglobin is too low, less oxygen is delivered to your body's cells and tissues, and you may feel tired or weak.

Anemia-related fatigue is experienced by more than three-fourths of all cancer patients. Over half of these patients report that fatigue associated with anemia affects the quality of their daily lives more than any other side effect of treatment, including nausea, pain, and depression. Most importantly, if left untreated, severe anemia can make cancer therapy less effective, interfere with the completion of chemotherapy, strain the heart and cardiovascular system, and result in the need for red blood cell transfusions.

Anemia in cancer patients can result from many factors, including chemotherapy, radiation treatment, blood loss, and iron deficiency. Cancer treatments are designed to destroy cancer cells but can also kill or damage healthy cells, including red blood cells that carry oxygen throughout the body. Chemotherapy can also suppress the production of red blood cells in the bone marrow and affect kidney function, including the production of *erythropoietin*, which stimulates red blood cell production.

## What Are the Symptoms of Anemia?

Anemia can be difficult to identify because early symptoms may be mild. If you're actively receiving treatment for cancer, you need to discuss with your oncologist or oncology nurse whether the treatment you're receiving affects your red blood cell count.

Report all symptoms of anemia to your doctor. Besides extreme fatigue and weakness, major symptoms of anemia can include:

- Shortness of breath
- Confusion or difficulty concentrating
- Dizziness or fainting
- Pale skin, including decreased pinkness of the lips, gums, lining of the eyelids, nail beds, and palms
- Rapid heartbeat
- Feeling cold
- Sadness or depression

Sometimes, patients are hesitant to tell their doctor how tired they are because they want the doctor to see them doing well; other times, patients simply associate fatigue with "being sick," assume it's a normal part of cancer treatment, or are fearful the cancer is worsening. As a part of being Patient Active in the management of anemia, you should be honest about the severity of your fatigue and its impact on your daily activities, and ask to have your blood counts tested. You shouldn't have to suffer unnecessarily.

## How Is Anemia Treated?

Doctors diagnose anemia with the help of a medical history and blood tests, including a complete blood count (CBC) to measure the number of red blood cells and the amount of hemoglobin in the blood. Normal hemoglobin ranges are 14–18 g/dL (grams per deciliter of blood) for men and 12–16 g/dL for women (Rogers et al.).

Treatment of anemia varies greatly depending upon the cause and extent of the condition. Your physician will help you determine the best treatment option for you. If your anemia is caused by chemotherapy, your doctor may prescribe injections of red blood cell growth factors to help you produce more red blood cells (Smith et al.). Ask your doctor which option will have the least impact on your daily activities and schedule. Once you're on the recommended treatment, let your healthcare team know whether you're getting any relief.

It's important to keep track of hemoglobin levels from your regular blood tests and compare them to your energy level. Discuss and share these observations with your medical team. Anemia-related fatigue is real. It shouldn't be ignored, as it can be treated. Talk with your doctor about what can be done to help improve your quality of life and keep your treatment on track.

## Pain

For many people, the scariest part of a cancer diagnosis is the fear of experiencing pain. But you should know that many people undergo cancer treatment without ever suffering from pain. Being Patient Active means knowing how to communicate about pain and how to take control of pain and discomfort effectively before you become distressed.

Cancer itself can cause pain in several different ways. People with cancer may have pain as a result of tumors pressing on an organ. In this case, pain may be relieved by using surgery to "debulk" (reduce the size or amount of) the tumor or by using radiation or chemotherapy to shrink it. Cancer can also cause pain when it spreads into the bones and damages their structure. Frequently, irradiating the bone relieves this type of pain. Pain can also occur when cancer presses on a nerve. This is often described as a burning, tingling, or shooting pain. Sometimes a nerve block, which makes the whole nerve numb, can be used to treat such a pain.

Unfortunately, cancer treatment itself can also cause pain and discomfort. Certain types of chemotherapy can cause *neuropathy* (numbness or tingling), which usually affects the hands or feet. Radiation or chemotherapy can cause damage to the lining of the esophagus or stomach (stomatitis), resulting in pain and discomfort.

In general, patients are frequently so concerned about taking too much medication and becoming addicted that they may not be getting adequate relief for pain. This common myth about pain management prevents many people from getting appropriate pain control. Poorly managed pain will increase anxiety and distress, which will in turn intensify feelings of pain. That's why it's important that you find a qualified professional who will work with you to break the cycle of pain and distress.

## Taking Control

First and foremost, talk to your doctor, nurse, and/or family about the pain or discomfort you are experiencing. Admitting that you are in pain is not a sign of weakness. Pain is a medical condition that can and should be treated. By talking about pain, you begin the process of controlling it.

Pain is hard to describe, but since you're the only one who can determine how much pain you're feeling, only you can effectively communicate it to your doctor or nurse. You can describe your pain in many ways. For example, you can use a number scale from zero to ten, with ten meaning the worst pain (see Pain Intensity Scale).

| Pain Intensity Scale | | | | | | | | | | |
|---|---|---|---|---|---|---|---|---|---|---|
| 0 | 1 | 2 | 3 | 4 | 5 | 6 | 7 | 8 | 9 | 10 |
| No Pain | | | | Medium Pain | | | | | Worst Pain | |

Once you and your doctor have identified the reason for your pain, the next step is usually choosing the correct medication. There may be a period of trial and error while your healthcare team tries to find the right medication and dosage for you. The many medications available range in strength and may be short-acting (lasting just a few hours) or long-acting (lasting twenty-four hours or more). Pain medications may be given as pills, liquids, suppositories, skin patches, or injections.

There have been many improvements in pain management, including patient-controlled analgesia systems, in which morphine or another type of medication is released when the patient presses a button. Usually non-narcotic medications, such as non-steroidal anti-inflammatory drugs, are used first. Pain that persists or increases is often treated with a combination of drugs and possibly a mild opiate, such as codeine. Stronger drugs, such as morphine, may be used if these other methods fail to be adequate.

For some people with cancer, certain non-drug pain treatments are effective. Mind-body practices such as guided imagery, relaxation and breathing exercises, biofeedback, massage, acupuncture, light exercise, music therapy, and counseling can help many people. Transcutaneous electrical nerve stimulation (TENS) units may also be used in specific circumstances. TENS involves giving small, non-painful electrical bursts to strategically located areas in the skin. Hot or cold packs may also provide relief from discomfort. *(See Chapter 7 for more on Complementary and Alternative Therapies.)*

Most patients will have complete relief of pain with appropriate management. You have a right to have your pain managed, but you need to communicate with your healthcare team about your symptoms. Pain is best managed when you work in partnership with your entire medical team. You can ask your oncologist to recommend a pain specialist if your pain is severe and previously tried treatments have not helped.

## What about Side Effects from Pain Medications?

Unfortunately, pain medication itself can cause side effects, including nausea, drowsiness, and constipation. Most people develop tolerance to the sedative effects of opioids, meaning that the medication may cause drowsiness at first, but it will eventually subside. Taking a stool softener or laxative—or a combination of both—can prevent constipation, another potential side effect of opioid pain medications.

Nausea may be treated with anti-nausea medication. If such solutions do not work, switching to a different pain medication may be necessary.

## Will I Become Addicted to Pain Medication?

People with cancer are frequently concerned about taking too much medication and "becoming addicted." This is a common myth about pain medicine that prevents many people from getting appropriate pain control. Addiction is the loss of control associated with taking a drug. Behaviors that characterize addiction include stealing drugs or money for drugs, lying to get them, and using drugs that are harmful. These are not the behaviors that people with cancer typically exhibit with regard to the medication needed for pain relief.

Addiction to pain medication is very rare in people with cancer. In fact, less than 1 percent of people with cancer who are treated with pain medication become addicted (Friedman). Poorly managed pain will increase anxiety and distress, which will in turn intensify feelings of pain. It's important that you find a qualified professional who can work with you to break the cycle of pain and distress. If you're struggling with controlling your pain, ask your doctor or nurse about how to find a pain specialist in your area.

### A Bill of Rights for People with Cancer Pain

1. I have the right to have my pain relieved by health professionals, family, friends, and others around me.
2. I have the right to have my pain controlled, no matter what its cause or how severe it may or may not be.
3. I have the right to be treated with respect at all times. When I need medication for pain, I shouldn't be treated like a drug abuser.
4. I have the right to have the pain resulting from treatments and procedures prevented or at least minimized (Rogers et al.).

## Rashes and Other Side Effects on the Skin

Besides hair loss, treatment toxicities of the skin range from rashes to redness and cracking to an acne-like eruption. Hyperpigmentation, or darkening of the skin, is another side effect seen with some chemotherapies and radiation treatments. The color changes can be seen in the nails, around intravenous infusion sites, the palms of the hands and soles of the feet, and, for some, a "tanning" all over the body.

Another effect, known as "hand and foot syndrome," causes a painful redness on the palms of the hands and soles of the feet. Sometimes this progresses to cracking and peeling. It's important to avoid heat or pressure in these areas to minimize the total effect. Other areas of pressure and resulting pain and redness are at the waistband and bra line. The use of water-based moisturizers is sometimes helpful in reducing the severity.

Skin rashes are sometimes seen with treatments. These can be small red bumps that are primarily located on the trunk of the body. Sometimes the rash gets severe enough that bumps merge, and the skin appears red over a large area. This rash can be itchy, painful, or develop pustules that can become infected. Many of the new biotherapies have skin side effects that can become quite severe. This acne-like rash is a result of the special way the new therapies work, but the rash can be serious. In fact, the risk of developing a serious skin infection is significant and must be managed carefully by your doctor.

Needless to say, the skin side effects of some treatments can be alarming and difficult to manage. However, you should follow your doctor's recommendations for management of any skin problems you may encounter and report the development of a rash to your doctor or nurse as soon as one develops. Continue protecting your skin from exposure to the sun by wearing sunscreen (if approved by your doctor), long-sleeved shirts and pants, and a hat. Treatments for cancer may increase your risk for skin sensitivities, and many skin problems are made worse by exposure to the sun.

### Blood-Clotting Problems

Keep track of your platelet count. If it falls below 20,000, or you notice any bruising, nosebleeds, or headaches, you are at risk for blood-clotting problems. Here's what to avoid:

- Don't take any medicine without first checking with your doctor or nurse. This includes aspirin or aspirin-free pain relievers (including acetaminophen, ibuprofen, and any other medicines you can buy without a prescription)
- Avoid alcoholic beverages
- Use a very soft toothbrush to clean your teeth
- Clean your nose by blowing gently into a soft tissue
- Take care not to cut or nick yourself when using scissors, needles, knives, or tools
- Be careful not to burn yourself when ironing or cooking. Use padded gloves when you reach into the oven
- Avoid contact sports and other activities that might result in injury

- Report any bleeding to your doctor immediately. You may need a platelet transfusion of red blood cells through an intravenous or central line in the outpatient clinic

## Gastrointestinal Side Effects

Nausea and vomiting are the side effects that most people associate with cancer treatment, but in the last fifteen years, great strides have been made in developing medications that have significantly decreased your chances of having major problems with these effects during your treatment. Your role in decreasing your chances of nausea and vomiting is to follow the medication instructions that you receive from your doctor or nurse, and consider some of these suggestions (Ettinger et al.):

- Eat only small, light meals before your treatment
- Eat several small meals during the day
- Dried toast, crackers, and cereal will help to settle your stomach
- Eat cool, bland foods (odors will trigger nausea)
- Avoid sweet, fatty, or fried foods
- Chew food slowly and well to help with digestion
- Drink liquids after meals to avoid feeling too full
- Use relaxation and slow, deep breathing to help manage any wave of nausea you might experience

Consult your doctor if nausea or vomiting becomes a problem. These symptoms can be managed, even if it takes trying several different combinations of medicines or therapeutic interventions.

## Constipation and Diarrhea

Difficulty having a bowel movement is common for people undergoing cancer treatment. Medications, surgery, inactivity, and dietary changes are just a few of the things that can contribute to changes in normal bowel function.

- Avoid over-the-counter stimulants to help you have a bowel movement
- Your doctor may suggest stool softeners or stool-softener-plus-laxative combinations to promote a normalization of movements. Another alternative would be to take fiber supplements, but this must be cleared with your doctor first

- Drink plenty of fluids (up to eight glasses of water a day) to help promote bowel function. Although fruit juices may be too sweet for you, consider preparing a drink of half-juice and half-water, or squeezing a lime or lemon into your water
- Try to avoid consuming many caffeinated beverages and sodas. For most patients, one drink each day with caffeine such as coffee, tea, or soda is okay, but remember that caffeine is a stimulant and interferes with your ability to relax and to sleep, increases your heart rate, causes diarrhea, decreases your appetite, and causes nausea. It may also cause you to feel nervous and jittery

Diarrhea is the passing of three or more watery bowel movements a day and can be a severe side effect of some cancer treatments. It's very important to manage this problem and get control of it quickly, because nutrients and body fluids are easily lost in a short period of time in this situation. If diarrhea is a side effect of your treatment, your healthcare team will discuss what to do, how to manage it, and when to call if it gets serious. Here's how to handle it:

- Drink plenty of fluids
- Eat six small meals a day
- Avoid greasy, fried, fatty foods
- Avoid foods high in acid, like tomatoes and citrus
- Consider a good, bland diet, such as the BRAT diet. BRAT is an acronym for bananas, rice, applesauce, and toast

As with other side effects of treatment, you should ask for clear instructions on how to take medications to prevent or manage diarrhea, when to phone the doctor for problems, and what to expect from your treatment. Try to keep track of your bowel movements by recording them because if the number increases to six or more, that's an indication that you should contact your doctor.

Practice good hygiene by washing your hands before and after going to the bathroom, wiping your bottom with a baby wipe or a mild soap and water, patting dry carefully, and applying an emollient ointment like zinc oxide or petroleum jelly afterward. Don't take any medication to control the diarrhea without consulting your doctor first.

Keeping track of the foods and situations that make any of these problems worse or better is helpful for you to manage your symptoms. Finding the right combinations of foods or mind-body interventions are some ways for you to take control of these side effects. You should write in your journal the things that work well for you and the things you need to avoid.

## Managing Gastric Upset with Good Nutrition

Nutrition is an integral part of maintaining good health through treatment and beyond. There are many resources from which you can make a plan to eat well and nutritiously; for example, most cancer clinics offer dietary consults for their patients.

You have read that six small meals are good for managing nausea and diarrhea. These meals should have adequate protein, carbohydrates, and fat to sustain your energy levels and assist in building your immune system and repairing your body. Consider alternatives to traditional meals, such as protein drinks or puddings. There are many vitamins and supplements that are available and sometimes even promoted to people with cancer. Be careful and a little wary of alternative therapies that boast impressive benefits. There are excellent resources available to help you practice caution and to be safe when considering these products—and your best resource is always to consult your healthcare team first.

## Other Side Effects

You may experience many other side effects during cancer treatment, including:

- Numbness
- Loss of appetite
- Mouth sores or gum and throat problems
- Rectal soreness
- Watery or dry eyes
- Bruising or bleeding
- Sexual concerns

If you're experiencing any of these side effects or have concerns about how you're feeling, be sure to write them down in your journal, and bring the journal with you to the doctor. You can also find more information about side effect management on our Web site at www. thewellnesscommunity.org or through the National Cancer Institute at www.cancer.gov.

Remember, you don't have to "tough it out" or pretend as if everything's all right. Cancer and its treatment bring profound challenges to you and your family. By taking charge of your treatment and any side effects you may be experiencing, you'll improve the quality of your life—and may well enhance the possibility of your recovery.

**Patient Action Plan**
- **Log any and all symptoms or side effects you may experience.**
  Report anything unusual to your doctor immediately
- **Immediately contact your doctor or nurse if your temperature is more than 100.4°F.**
  You may have to go to the hospital for medication and hydration
- **Identify needs, and ask for help.**
  Family, friends, neighbors, and members of your religious community may be able to help with chores and errands, such as transportation, grocery shopping, walking the dog, weeding the garden, and housework
- **Practice energy conservation.**
  Learn to prioritize, pace yourself, ask others for help, eliminate unnecessary tasks, modify how you do things, and avoid things that cause stress
- **Keep track of your hemoglobin levels, and compare them with your energy levels.**
  Discuss and share these observations with your healthcare team

## Chapter 10

# Managing Practical Matters

*I'm frustrated with the insurance company's power to dictate the hospital for which they will approve surgeries—yet I am grateful that I have insurance. I've received no bills and have been able to eliminate all consumer debt because of supplemental (AFLAC) insurance offered by my employer. I'm also taking early withdrawal on my 401k.*

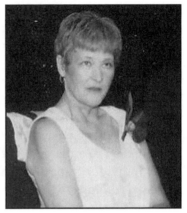

—Louise Carole,
*participant, The Wellness Community - Orange County*

WHILE THE THOUGHTS OF cancer patients primarily center on health and recovery issues, concerns related to finances, insurance, legal issues, and employment usually follow closely behind. Although most people in this country have some sort of health insurance coverage, many cancer patients fear that the illness will drain their family's financial reserves, wonder whether they'll be able to continue to work or return to work, and what insurance coverage protections are guaranteed by law.

## Health Insurance

Health insurance coverage provides assistance with medical expenses involved in screening, diagnosing, treating, and recovering from illness. You should investigate the terms of your policy to be aware of the provisions for hospital stays, special or experimental treatments, second opinions, diagnostic measures, and long-term and/or home care. Some policies may cover nursing services or alternative healthcare services. Knowledge of any restrictions in the healthcare coverage will help avoid disappointment and unpaid medical bills.

The healthcare insurance industry has been in a constant state of change for the last ten years as different types of managed care plans replace the traditional indemnity insurance that covered whichever doctor and hospital the patient visited.

Most laws governing these health-insurance companies are determined by individual states and vary widely in different regions of the country. The recent addition of for-profit healthcare conglomerates has added to the ever more confusing picture. Currently, many rules governing Medicare, Medicaid, and "third-party payers" are under review at the state and national levels.

A relatively new term and concept in healthcare is *case management*, which refers to a planned approach to manage services and treatments for an individual's specific healthcare needs. The goal is to provide effective interventions to meet these needs while containing costs.

There's been much controversy recently about access to treatment for cancer patients. While all of us are concerned about controlling healthcare costs, no one wants to be denied access to appropriate testing or treatments. If payment is denied, it's best for you to work with your doctor and/or treatment facility in order to reapply for appropriate payments.

If these efforts fail, there are a number of reimbursement specialists that operate hotlines for various drug manufacturers—and several may even contact the insurance company directly on your behalf.

Patient advocates, lawyers, the patient, and/or a family member can also pursue claim rejections with insurers and, sometimes after a long and arduous battle, obtain payment. If all else fails, contacting your local state legislator may provide the necessary clout to gain pre-approval for a needed test or treatment.

## Types of Health Insurance

*Health Maintenance Organizations* (*HMOs*) provide, offer, or arrange for a wide range of healthcare services to cover a specified group of enrollees for a fixed, periodic prepayment. With an HMO, all costs are covered—sometimes with minimum co-pay—as long as an appropriate

referral is obtained before seeking any care outside of the office of the primary provider. However, it may be difficult to obtain coverage for second or third opinions or treatment from a healthcare provider who is not part of that particular HMO system.

*Indemnity insurance policies* are the traditional insurances in which physicians and other providers receive payment based on each billing charge for a visit or service provided. While indemnity policies provide the best coverage in terms of flexibility, there is usually a deductible and/or co-pay required for doctor visits and medications.

*Preferred Provider Organizations* (PPOs) combine some aspects of the HMO and the traditional indemnity policies. The patient may choose his or her provider from a list of "preferred providers" and does not need a referral before seeking additional opinions or treatment. However, if you make a decision to see a provider or seek hospitalization in a center outside the network, the co-pay is significant.

*Major medical* is a plan that is usually part of the traditional indemnity insurance that pays for a percentage of expenses not covered by the hospitalization part of the plan.

*Medicare, Medicaid,* and *veterans benefits*: Medicare, a federal insurance program, provides coverage for testing, hospitalization, and treatments for people age sixty-five or older. Medicaid is a joint federal and state health insurance program and provides coverage for some low-income and disabled people. People with Medicare or Medicaid coverage are usually offered managed care or indemnity (traditional) coverage plans, depending on the state in which they live. Veterans may receive benefits through the Veterans Affairs program, in addition to whatever coverage they may have under other insurance programs.

*COBRA*, or the *Consolidated Omnibus Budget Reconciliation Act*, is a federal law that allows a person to maintain insurance coverage. A person may continue to be covered by his or her last employer's insurance for up to eighteen months, but he or she is responsible for paying the monthly premiums.

Short- and long-term *disability insurance* may provide financial assistance when a person is being treated for cancer. An employer may carry disability insurance for employees, and/or an individual may purchase policies from private insurance carriers.

There are two different disability benefits available from the Social Security Administration: *Social Security Disability Insurance* (*SSDI*) and

*Supplemental Security Income (SSI)*. The medical requirements and determination process is the same under both programs. Eligibility for Social Security Disability is based on your work history and begins six months after you are considered disabled. For people younger than sixty-five, Medicare health coverage doesn't begin for twenty-four months. SSI disability payments are made on the basis of financial need, and most people who get SSI are also eligible for food stamps and Medicaid.

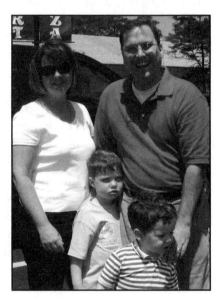

*I remember thinking [upon diagnosis] that if I were to die, I would be denied the opportunity to watch my children grow up and that all the plans and dreams my wife and I had would have to go unfulfilled. Every thought I had was worse and more tragic than the last. However, even in those first few moments, one thought was able to penetrate my burgeoning sadness and provide solace and peace of mind: Though I may die, and my wife and children be emotionally devastated, at least my life insurance will assure that their lives are not destroyed.*

—Drew Van Dopp,
*participant, The Wellness Community - Delmarva*

**Obtaining Adequate Life Insurance**
The following suggestions from *Charting The Journey: An Almanac of Practical Resources for Cancer Survivors* by the National Coalition for Cancer Survivorship may increase a cancer survivor's ability to obtain adequate life insurance:
- Try large companies that carefully grade type and stage of cancer
- Obtain estimates from several companies. An efficient way to do this is to have an independent agent (one who does not work for a particular company) shop among the

companies in your area to obtain the best possible plan for your needs. You may get a list of all licensed insurance brokers in your area from the state insurance department

- If you are unable to obtain a life-insurance policy with full death benefits, consider a graded policy. If you die from cancer within the first few years of the policy— usually three years—a graded policy returns only your premium plus part of the face value of the policy to your beneficiaries. If you die after the waiting period has passed, the company will pay the full face of the policy

- Try to obtain life insurance through a group plan. Many employers and organizations that offer group health insurance also offer group life insurance. The insurance company does not make an individual evaluation of the health of each plan member of a large group; however, your health may be considered if you participate in a plan with a small number of members (for example, if you are one of thirty workers). If your health is considered, you may be excluded from the plan, denied full benefits, or required to pay an extra premium

The American Council on Life Insurance (1001 Pennsylvania Avenue, NW, Washington, DC 20004) provides information about brokers who specialize in high-risk life insurance.

## Viatical Settlements

A viatical settlement is an option in which the patient sells his or her life insurance policy for a percentage of the total face value. This enables you to receive a sizable sum of money to be used entirely at your own discretion. By selling a life insurance policy to a company that specializes in providing viatical settlements, you can obtain cash quickly and easily at a time when you may need the most financial help.

## Employment and Legal Issues

While many people with cancer feel unable to continue with their normal employments during treatment, some people find that maintaining as much of their "normal" lifestyles as possible is extremely valuable. If you feel able to work, there's probably no reason why you shouldn't be able to do so.

*The Americans with Disabilities Act (ADA)* is a relatively new law that redefines disabilities to include cancer. Under the act, anyone who has had cancer is considered disabled. The goal of the ADA is to end job discrimination against people with disabilities, including discrimination regarding hiring, promotions, firing, pay, job training, and other aspects of work including job benefits. A booklet from the American Cancer Society, *Americans With Disability Act: Legal Protection for Cancer Patients Against Employment Discrimination,* provides a comprehensive overview of how you might be protected by this law.

*The Family and Medical Leave Act* allows a patient or a family member caring for an ill person to take up to twelve weeks off from work, without pay but without loss of benefits.

Many cancer survivors need some physical rehabilitation before they are able to return to their old jobs or start new ones. Several different kinds of physical rehabilitation that might be helpful include: physical therapy to gain strength and mobility, occupational therapy to increase strength and coordination of the body and to evaluate the ability to return to daily activities, and rehabilitation counseling to help deal with the emotional impact of disability.

Employment rehabilitation may be needed if you decide to seek a different kind of work than you did before cancer. You may be eligible for job retraining through the *Vocational Rehabilitation Act* of 1973, and there are employment agencies that can help with this process. The Office of Vocational Rehabilitation or a private employment agency can assist you in finding out about these services.

*The Wellness Community changed my life from one of loneliness and despair to one of hope and compassion. I believe that cancer is not just a physical disease, but one that affects and consumes every facet of life. I went from a wealthy businesswoman to a woman with no income, hoping to qualify for disability while I regroup and redefine what wellness is for me.*

—JUDITH TARBELL,
*participant, The Wellness Community - Orange County*

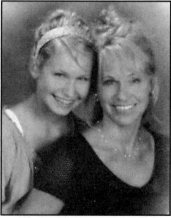

Judith Tarbell, far right

## Seeking Legal Assistance

If you feel you've experienced discrimination in employment or insurance matters, you may decide to seek the advice of an attorney. In this case, it's highly advisable to contact a lawyer who specializes in employment or insurance law and has experience working with people who've had cancer.

*Lawyer referral services* are programs provided by a local or state bar association and are designed to help you locate a private attorney to handle legal matters or problems. There may be a fee for the first consultation. The referral service may be able to help you decide whether you need to see a lawyer.

If you need a lawyer but can't afford legal fees, a useful resource is the legal aid or legal services office in your county of residence. These offices handle some types of legal matters for people eligible under income guidelines established for their operation.

## Important Papers

While most people with cancer recover and live for many years after their initial treatments, fears about declining health may stimulate thoughts about wills and living wills. People have a legal and moral right to decide what kind of medical treatment they want or don't want if and when they are seriously ill and their deaths are expected. They have a right to choose who will make decisions for them when they are no longer able to speak or think clearly and to designate who will get their property after they die.

A *will* is a legal document, usually prepared with the assistance of a lawyer, which designates the distribution of a person's property after his or her death. This document determines who will get the person's money and belongings and who will be responsible for a person's underage children in the absence of the other parent. In many states, if there's no will, an agent of the state will make these decisions.

An *advance directive* is a general term that refers to your oral and written instructions about your future medical care, in the event that you become unable to speak for yourself. Each state regulates the use of advance directives differently. There are two types of advance directives: a living will and a medical power of attorney.

A *living will* is a type of advance directive prepared by an individual that puts in writing his or her wishes concerning medical treatment if a time should come when he or she is no longer able to express those wishes verbally. Most states honor a living will prepared in advance by a patient; however, the laws concerning the preparation and implementation of such a document vary from state to state.

A *medical power of attorney* is a document that enables you to appoint someone you trust to make decisions about your medical care if you cannot make those decisions yourself. This type of advance directive may also be called a "healthcare proxy" or "appointment of a healthcare agent." The person you appoint may be called your healthcare agent, surrogate, attorney-in-fact, or proxy.

In many states, the person you appoint through a medical power of attorney is authorized to speak for you any time you are unable to make your own medical decisions, not just at the end of life. It's important to choose the person who's most likely to be able to carry out your wishes; sometimes a spouse or close family member may not be the best one because he or she is too emotionally involved. Be sure your proxy or agent has access to the signed directives and that your oncologist has a copy, as well.

When it comes to handling practical matters, discussing all of your decisions with close family members, supportive friends, spiritual advisors, and healthcare providers will minimize confusion and help everyone involved feel more comfortable with whatever decisions you make.

### Patient Action Plan

- Review your insurance policy to become familiar with what kind of policy it is and what it covers
- Keep careful records of all expenses related to medical treatment, even transportation, because major medical insurance may cover expenses not covered by the hospitalization plan. Uncovered medical expenses are tax deductible if they exceed a certain percentage of your adjusted gross income
- Fill out any required claim forms, and file as promptly as possible. If needed, seek help in filling out forms from the doctor's office, the hospital social worker, or the home-care agency
- Keep copies of everything submitted, as well as all claims that have been paid
- Follow up with the insurance company with any questions about filed claims

- If your medical and other bills begin to accumulate faster than you can pay them, don't wait for a crisis—approach your creditors to work out a payment schedule you can manage
- Consider your insurance needs if you wish to change jobs, and do not give up the insurance you have until you have determined where you will obtain future coverage
- Do not allow your insurance to expire
- Work with an experienced attorney to draft your will and advance directives, including your living will and medical power of attorney

# Part Three

# Making the Mind-Body-Spirit Connection

## Chapter 11

# Living with Cancer

*I'm certainly more humble. I'm mellow, not wearing my feelings on my sleeve, not thinking everything has to be my way. I don't take myself or others too seriously. I express myself differently and am more in touch with God. I laugh more, love more, and feel more. Life matters.*

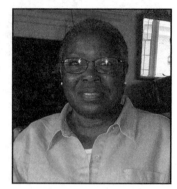

—ALICE JUNE TRIBBLE,
*participant, The Wellness Community -
Greater Cincinnati/Northern Kentucky*

ESPITE PROGRESS IN THE early detection and treatment of many cancers, the diagnosis of cancer can instill fear and anxiety in a patient. Cancer can disrupt daily life, including family, work, education, friendships, and finances. Research has shown in general that 25–30 percent of newly diagnosed and recurrent patients experience elevated levels of emotional distress, while as many as 47 percent have a psychiatric diagnosis (Marcus).

Sometimes, the type and severity of the cancer and/or its treatment can create emotional distress for the individual with cancer and his or her loved ones. For example, a study published in 2001 reported that people with lung cancer, as a group, experienced the highest levels of emotional distress, followed by people with brain tumors or pancreatic cancer. This study and others demonstrate the need for support services for people with cancer and underscores the need for psychosocial screening to determine the level of distress and risk of emotional difficulties for people with cancer. Just as scientists are working to discover how to detect cancer earlier, psychosocial oncology professionals would like to help identify emotional distress or other psychosocial concerns early on in your diagnosis so that you can get the support you need to actively participate in treatment and maintain a good quality of life throughout cancer and beyond.

## What Is Distress?

First and foremost, distress has many different dimensions. It's not easily described as one single emotional or physical reaction. Distress, as it relates to a person with cancer, focuses on describing or measuring the unpleasant emotional experiences that can impact cognitive, behavioral, social, emotional, and spiritual functioning and may also interfere with the person's ability to cope effectively with cancer, its physical symptoms, and its treatment.

Distress extends along a continuum, ranging from common feelings of vulnerability, sadness, and fears to problems that can become more disabling, such as depression, anxiety, panic, social isolation, and existential and spiritual crisis.

According to the National Comprehensive Cancer Network's (NCCN) Distress Management Guidelines, "Distress should be recognized, monitored, documented, and treated promptly at all stages of disease. All patients should be screened for distress at their initial visit, at appropriate intervals, and as clinically indicated especially with changes in disease status (remission, recurrence, progression). Screening should identify the level and nature of the distress. Distress should be assessed and managed according to clinical practice guidelines."

Jimmie Holland, M.D., and her colleagues have developed and researched a simple tool, called the *Distress Thermometer*, to measure distress, in order to help people with cancer, their caregivers, and healthcare professionals better determine and effectively treat their distress. The Distress Thermometer asks you to quantify on a scale of zero to ten your global level of distress during the past week, including the day you complete the survey. A score of four or higher for any item flags a significant level of distress that suggests it would be helpful to seek support from your healthcare team. In addition, you can also identify specific parts of your life that have caused you distress during the past week. The tool contains thirty-three items, divided into five broad categories that include practical problems, family problems, emotional problems, spiritual/religious concerns, and physical problems.

### Distress-Measuring Tool

Instructions: In the chart, first please circle the number (0–10) that best describes how much distress you have been experiencing in the past week, including today. Second, please indicate below if any of the following has been a problem for you in the past week, including today. Be sure to check YES or NO for each.

0  1  2  3  4  5  6  7  8  9  10

| YES | NO | PRACTICAL PROBLEMS | YES | NO | PHYSICAL PROBLEMS |
|-----|-----|-----|-----|-----|-----|
| O | O | Child care | O | O | Appearance |
| O | O | Housing | O | O | Bathing/dressing |
| O | O | Insurance | O | O | Breathing |
| O | O | Transportation | O | O | Changes in urination |
| O | O | Work/school | O | O | Constipation |
| YES | NO | FAMILY PROBLEMS | O | O | Eating |
| O | O | Dealing with children | O | O | Diarrhea |
| O | O | Dealing with partner | O | O | Fatigue |
| YES | NO | EMOTIONAL PROBLEMS | O | O | Feeling swollen |
| O | O | Depression | O | O | Fevers |
| O | O | Fears | O | O | Getting around |
| O | O | Nervousness | O | O | Indigestion |
| O | O | Sadness | O | O | Mouth sores |
| O | O | Worry | O | O | Nausea |
| O | O | Sexual | O | O | Nose dry/congested |
| YES | NO | SPIRITUAL/RELIGIOUS CONCERNS | O | O | Pain |
| O | O | Loss of faith | O | O | Skin dry/itchy |
| O | O | Relating to God | O | O | Sleep |
| O | O | Loss of meaning or purpose of life | O | O | Tingling in hands/feet |

Other Problems:

*Source: Jimmie Holland, M.D.*

## Dealing with Feelings of Depression

People dealing with cancer may experience a wide range of emotions—from anger, joy, and hope to sadness and despair.

Sometimes crying and expressing your sadness can be enough to get you through the tough emotions that can come with your diagnosis. But sometimes you may feel so bad that you lose interest in the things that used to make you happy. You may feel like staying in bed all day, and stop reaching out to friends and family, preferring to be alone in your misery.

If you start feeling this way, you may be suffering from the psychological condition called *depression.* Depression and emotional distress can make it more difficult for you to cope with the physical symptoms from your cancer and your treatment. Long-term distress, including depression and intense anxiety, might even affect your immune system, making it harder for your body to fight illness. Many people with cancer experience some degree of depression, but thankfully, there are also many highly effective treatments for this condition.

The first and most important step in treating depression is to recognize that it's a problem and ask for help. If you think you may be suffering from depression, talk to your doctor or to a social worker or professional counselor. Tell him or her how you're feeling so he or she can help you figure out what might make you feel better.

## Handling the Pressure

People with cancer and their family members are under a great deal of pressure to cope rationally and effectively with the treatments, side effects, and anxieties that accompany the diagnosis. Every single patient, at every stage of disease, regardless of the type of treatment, deals with issues that cause some level of distress (Marcus; Benjamin).

The psychological impact of cancer can vary considerably among individuals, depending on the extent of the disease and each personal situation and personality. Living with cancer and undergoing treatment can affect someone's ability to lead his or her usual lifestyle and may cause changes in family roles, a depletion of financial resources, and a decrease in self-esteem (Derogatis et al.). At The Wellness Community, people with cancer learn that, by working together, they can overcome the most common emotional concerns associated with cancer.

Although emotional distress is common, it is frequently an ignored side effect of cancer. Many people are hesitant to share their concerns for fear that others will see them as "weak" or not having a "positive attitude." In fact, it's normal for people who are dealing with cancer to experience a whole range of emotions.

Emotional distress can range from common feelings of vulnerability, sadness, and fear of recurrence or death to problems that are more disabling, such as clinical depression, intense anxiety, or panic. Emotional distress can affect your ability to carry out daily activities and to participate actively in your treatment. It can also make physical symptoms more severe or even impact the treatment outcome.

Side effects from cancer treatment can add to the emotional distress that you and your family experience. When side effects interfere with daily activities or disrupt treatment schedules, you might become even more anxious and afraid that you won't be able to cope with the rigors of treatment. Treatment side effects and psychological well-being should be addressed simultaneously to maximize your ability to cope and recover, both physically and emotionally, from cancer.

It takes time to accept the diagnosis of cancer and to understand what it will mean for both you and your family. Everyone's reactions will differ and will probably vary over time. But you're not alone. Many other people with cancer share these feelings and concerns, and sometimes it helps to talk with other people going through treatment. By becoming Patient Active, you can regain a sense of control about your treatment and your life, and you can find hope and meaning throughout the cancer experience.

## What Are the Stages of Emotional Distress?

While emotional reactions to the diagnosis, treatment, and side effects of cancer may vary widely, some responses are quite common. Before you get your first treatment, you may feel that no one understands what you're going through. It is important at this time to gather as much information as possible and to find someone to talk to who has been through treatment.

By the middle of treatment, you may feel overwhelmed, even unable to manage daily responsibilities. This is a normal reaction and often reflects the strain on your physical and emotional energy as you manage treatment and cope with your situation.

Upon completing treatment, you may feel abandoned by your healthcare team or other supportive people who were involved during treatment, or you may feel anxious about the cancer returning. Throughout this time, you and your caregivers may find that a support group can be beneficial in learning valuable information and feeling less alone in making the transition from being ill to living well after cancer.

Anger is also a normal and healthy response to having cancer. It is an emotion that may arise during interactions with members of the healthcare system or your own family. If you, like many other people, were raised to view expressions of anger as wrong, you may feel guilty and try to deny these feelings. However, expressing anger in a productive and thoughtful manner can prevent emotions from building up and potentially leading to more serious emotional problems such as hostility, irresponsibility, and inconsiderate impulses.

### Finding a Way to COPE

According to the *Journal of Psychosocial Oncology*, the COPE model, based on an orderly problem-solving approach, is a useful tool for when you experience psychological distress. Here's how it works:

**C:** Creativity in problem-solving; can be achieved with brainstorming

**O:** Optimism, or staying focused on the positive

**P:** Planning manageable ways to deal with your emotions

**E:** Expert information, which you should do you best to locate whenever you need it

## Stress and the Immune System

*Psychoneuroimmunology (PNI)* is a recent scientific discipline that studies the link between the mind and the body—how thoughts, feelings, and attitudes positively or negatively affect illness or health. The Wellness Community program links the findings from PNI with its application to psychosocial support. From the beginning, TWC's Patient Active

Concept and program has been rooted in the application of the findings from psychoneuroimmunology.

In this area of PNI, scientists propose that long-term unremitting stress reduces or diminishes the positive impact of the immune system, while positive emotions enhance the immune system. Because the first line of defense against illness or disease progression is the immune system, enhancing its power by reducing stress and increasing positive emotions—at the very least—improves your quality of life and may even enhance the possibility of recovery.

### Other Stress-Reducing Techniques

There appear to be several ways to cope actively with cancer that not only improve quality of life, but may actually enhance immune function. These include:

- Managing stress through muscle relaxation, mindfulness meditation, or other stress reduction methods
- Problem-solving strategies, especially with difficult treatment decisions
- Managing side effects of treatment—especially fatigue and pain
- Managing lingering depression, and making sure that it is treated

In thinking about this possibility and, especially, the notion of enhancing the power of the immune system by reducing stress, several questions immediately come to mind:

- What are your most significant stressors?
- Which emotions are positive and should be boosted?
- Which are negative and should be diminished?
- Which stressors should be reduced?

*In the past year, I've progressed...to a degree of acceptance and a sense of community with others. Fears remain, of course, but they're much easier to deal with through the open exchange with others who are in similar circumstances...and they're diminished by the knowledge that together we can find strength. Our friends have become like family as we proceed toward recovery.*

—Virginia L. Moore,
*participant, The Wellness Community - Central Arizona*

## The Expression of Emotions

Another new discovery in cancer relates to important research on emotional expression. This research has been applied to people participating in cancer support groups and professionally facilitated support groups similar to those offered at TWC. Over the last twenty-five years, psychosocial oncology has aimed to incorporate new research findings into the way programs and services for emotional support are delivered.

Through psychosocial oncology research, oncology professionals have learned that the expression of emotions is an important component for managing the diagnosis and treatment of cancer. In particular, primary negative emotions—fear, anger, and sadness— are normal and adaptive. Research has shown that the process of accessing, expressing, integrating, and reframing your emotions within a support group improves *quality of life*. However, if these same emotions are repressed, they can lead to aggressiveness, hostility, and irresponsible and inconsiderate impulses.

Restraining hostile, impulsive, irresponsible, and thoughtless behavior is positively associated with improved quality of life, lower levels of distress, and better social functioning (Giese-Davis). Restraint should not be confused with suppressing your emotions; suppressing emotions is associated with negative mental health.

> **For Better Health, Express Yourself**
> Learning to express a whole range of emotions within a support group can lead to:
> - Decreases in hostility
> - Greater self-confidence and assertion
> - Greater expressions of support, empathy, interest, and humor
> - Better physical health and physiological functioning (Greenberg et al.)
>
> Honing these skills may enable you to balance the expression of strong emotions without alienating others—especially family and friends (Giese-Davis).

*I went from working a lot to being on disability.... That is a 100 percent change. The cancer stopped me from hunting—something I loved—and stopped me from doing my own housework.*

—KARL M. JACKSON,
*participant and TWC Medal of Courage winner,*
*The Wellness Community - Philadelphia*

## The Challenge of the "Positive Attitude"

People with cancer have long been told that having a positive attitude increases their chances of survival. But how true is this? Is it really all that important to have a positive attitude in order to battle cancer and improve outcomes? And conversely, will a negative attitude mean a worse outcome or earlier death? The answer to both questions is: not necessarily.

In a 2004 study by Penelope Schofield and her colleagues at Peter Mac-Callum Cancer Centre in Melbourne, Australia, that involved 204 lung cancer patients, there was *no evidence* that a high level of optimism prior to treatment enhanced survival. However, the study underscored the importance of optimism in relation to *quality of life. Those patients who were more optimistic were less depressed and more likely to adhere to treatment.*

Another new body of work goes beyond just looking at a positive attitude and is examining its biological underpinnings by studying immune function and stress hormones. So far, the findings are similar to the Schofield study, indicating that successful coping is not necessarily about having a positive outlook or striving for a cheery disposition. *Rather, coping in a way familiar to you, which could involve anything from stress relief to exercise, can prove to be beneficial.* In fact, if you're a natural curmudgeon, then continuing to be a curmudgeon may be the very thing to help lower stress, bolster the immune system, and, possibly, influence the success of your cancer treatment (Marcus).

This new research doesn't just focus on patients' tendencies to look at the glass as half-full or half-empty and how those attitudes may influence survival outcomes. Researchers are also examining *how different coping styles may affect biological indicators of disease-fighting ability* such as *cortisol* rhythms (measures of stress levels) and natural killer cell counts (measures of immune response). With better understanding of these biological variables, there may be ways (such as muscle relaxation, stress reduction exercises, or problem solving) to help patients maintain stress and natural killer cells at levels that improve their chances of extending survival.

For instance, researchers are measuring cortisol levels in women's saliva and counting white blood cells to determine if there is a connection between cortisol levels and the immune system. In an ongoing study, preliminarily published in 2000 in the *Journal of the National Cancer Institute*, researchers found that patients whose cortisol levels were flat and didn't follow the typical pattern of decline throughout the day died sooner than women with normal, fluctuating cortisol patterns. The finding, researchers believe, indicates that a psychological intervention may boost one's disease-fighting ability, a notion that in the past has driven the focus on staying positive.

Researchers are now realizing that people cope with stress in vastly different ways. *Individuals need to identify solutions that match their natural temperaments and personalities.* The next step is finding the mechanisms that enable patients to keep their cortisol patterns and natural killer cells at optimum levels and, hopefully, extend their survival. For some patients, this may happen by being uncooperative and unpleasant rather than positive, if this is their normal coping strategy toward stress.

For example, at Ohio State University, an ongoing study is measuring not only survival rates but also endocrine responses and biological markers of immunity. Women participating in the study, all of whom share similar diagnoses of breast cancer, are learning muscle relaxation, problem-solving, and time-management techniques. They are making dietary changes, such as reducing fat intake, increasing fiber, and exercising, all in the hope that some methods will bolster the women's ability to fight and, ultimately, beat the disease (Marcus).

In essence, people with cancer should be encouraged to *develop realistic expectations about their illness so they can make good decisions about their care and not be pressured to be blindly positive.* The important distinction is that optimism should not exclude sadness, anger, sorrow, grief, and hurt. You can decide to go on in the face of all of that, knowing the outcome isn't under your control.

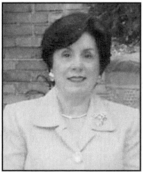

*I believe that my encounter with this disease was a blessing in many ways, helping me to see what's really important in life: the love of your family, the simple pleasures of being alive, the beauty in nature, and meeting many wonderful people that I never would've known, who've become landmarks along my journey. As a result, I volunteer at TWC of Central New Jersey and at the American Cancer Society.*

—CHRISTINE SALEMI,
*participant, The Wellness Community - Central New Jersey*

## Is There a Difference Between Optimism and Hope?

Jerome Groopman, M.D., author of *The Anatomy of Hope*, elaborates on the above idea by explaining that a positive attitude, or optimism, is the thought that "everything is going to turn out for the best." But life isn't like that. Sometimes bad things happen to wonderful people. Hope, in contrast, doesn't make that assumption but rather, in a clear-eyed manner, assesses all the problems, challenges, or obstacles. Through information and education, the hopeful person seeks and finds a possible realistic path to a better future—a future that is often unknown and unknowable but is constantly reassessed based upon new information. A person with true hope will experience a wide range of emotions, including fear, anger, and sadness and will try to move forward through all the difficulties (Groopman).

At The Wellness Community, we understand hope to be something participants gain from each other. After all, there's no person a cancer patient would rather see than a cancer survivor. The ability to make pragmatic decisions in the face of cancer based upon being with others who know what you're going through is an essential ingredient at TWC. Participants learn from each other and can increase hope, as well as reduce some of the stress associated with cancer (Benjamin). If longer survival is not possible, then it's reasonable to hope for other meaningful outcomes—like hoping for a peaceful death or the resolution of family conflicts. Gaining information and support from others with cancer may lead to positive immunological and stress hormone responses.

**Patient Action Plan**
- **Depression is a medical condition.**
  It is a condition associated with a chemical imbalance in your brain. There are medications that can restore the balance and make you feel better
- **Admitting that you're depressed does not mean that you're weak or that you're a whiner or complainer.**
  Depression is a very serious condition and you should not try to deal with it on your own. It takes courage and strength to admit that you need help and to get treatment
- **Recognize the link between stress and the immune system.**
  It's important to tell your doctor if you have feelings of depression and emotional distress. Your healthcare team is there to help you cope with these feelings, and to

make sure that they do not have a negative impact on your immune system

- **Express your emotions in a healthier manner**.
  Find creative new ways to reduce your stress levels
- **Getting treated for depression can make a huge difference in your quality of life**.
  You have enough to handle when you have cancer without also being clinically depressed. Relieving the depression will make it easier to deal with everything else and will allow you to rediscover joys and pleasures in your everyday life

## Chapter 12

# It's Not Just You
## Cancer Is a "Family" Disease

*There are only four kinds of people in the world:*
*Those who have been caregivers;*
*Those who are currently caregivers;*
*Those who will be caregivers; and*
*Those who will need caregivers.*

—ROSALYNN CARTER,
*Helping Yourself Help Others*

WHILE RELAXATION CAN WORK wonders in helping to manage stress and side effects, nothing helps more than a strong support system. If you're blessed with close, loving caregivers and allow them to do their work to help you throughout your cancer experience, you can and will find the strength to keep going.

Research shows that people who are well connected to others have a lower death rate from all causes or diseases; those who completely isolate themselves have the highest mortality rates. Therefore, connecting with caregivers as early as possible in the treatment process obviously offers a better prognosis.

But who are your caregivers? In many cases, these are the people you've known and loved your whole life. They can be spouses, close friends, neighbors, or even complete strangers. Meeting new people who have been where you are at this moment in time can be of tremendous help, and such meaningful interaction is the basis of support groups. No one else in the world understands the cancer experience as honestly and completely as others who are in the same situation. Some groups are for cancer patients and their families, while others are limited to patients or caregivers only. *(For more on how to network with a support group, see Chapter 14.)*

If you're a person with cancer, this chapter is for you, but it also contains "Caregiver's Corner" sections for your caregiver, because the journey toward wellness is not meant to be traveled alone. If it takes a village to raise a child, it certainly takes a community of caring people to help a patient through an illness as challenging as cancer.

## Don't Let Family and Friends Abandon You

As unbelievable as it may seem, sometimes family and friends abandon people with cancer. That abandonment can be physical (i.e., staying away) or emotional (i.e., distant, distracted, or unavailable). None of these responses to cancer are unusual, but let's look at how you can avoid unwanted loneliness, because that's an unpleasant situation that can literally depress your immune system.

If you've experienced a significant change in your relationships since your diagnosis—if your friends and family seem more distant than before—it's probably not because they don't love you anymore. It's much more likely that they are simply uncomfortable around people with cancer, feeling inadequate or unable to say or do "the right thing."

### Reasons Family and Friends May Seem Distant
- They can't bear to be with someone they love when that person is suffering and, perhaps in their minds, ultimately doomed
- Being with the person who has cancer reminds them of their own vulnerability and mortality
- They can only think about the illness and, yet, are afraid to utter the word "cancer," especially in the presence of a loved one with cancer
- They want to help but feel inadequate or helpless themselves
- They have an irrational fear that cancer is somehow contagious
- They are afraid they can't deal with the cancer patient's honesty about his or her situation, or that they won't be able to bear it themselves

At The Wellness Community, we've all watched cancer patients become more and more isolated simply because they have cancer. But we suggest two ways of reaching out for the social support you need. First, talk to your friends and family directly and openly about the subject of your cancer. Ask for their help, and remind them that, although you have cancer now, you want the relationship to go on as it's always been. Second, ask your family and friends how you've changed since your diagnosis. Maybe there's something different about you that's causing them to stay away from you.

Chances are, your friends and family don't want to abandon you at all. They just don't know how to talk or act with you now—and they may find this reaction frightening. Talking with you just as openly as they used to will go a long way toward helping them work through their fears—and will best help them to start helping you.

## Create a "Circle of Care"

You've probably said to yourself many times: "No one understands exactly what I'm going through right now." But how can others even begin to understand unless you involve them every step of the way?

Think about the people closest to you. Who has the personal strengths on which you feel you can rely, in good times and bad? For instance, your spouse may be best at providing emotional strength, while your sister or brother may be better suited for gathering the latest cancer news and research. Or maybe you have adult children who can help as *communicators* who keep everyone else in your life informed and connected, especially in times when you can't or don't feel like talking. The important thing is to let all of those around you help in the ways they feel they can contribute the most.

Many of The Wellness Community participants have created their own "circles of care" with several family members taking an active role in the various aspects of their treatments and well-being. You can easily do the same. Rely on this support system to help you navigate your way through the decision-making process; ask for advice and listen to the concerns, input, and feedback of all involved. Allowing your family members to participate in this manner will empower them to help you more than you ever dreamed possible—and such a positive experience can only enhance your own well-being. It's healthiest for you to have support!

*I think getting the whole family involved as soon as possible can really help to take the edge off of things. We told all five of our kids about David's diagnosis as soon as we knew, and although they were all over the country, they immediately mobilized and asked what they could do. We got calls before, during, and after each treatment, and it helped so much to know that this was a disease we were all dealing with together.*

—JOAN FRIEDER,
*participant, The Wellness Community - Philadelphia*

## Creative Ways to Let Your Family Help

Dealing with cancer can be overwhelming for both you and your primary caregiver, and you may quickly discover that a little help can go a long way. Of course, once you're in the middle of treatments, you may be too exhausted to ask for help. That's why it makes very good sense to put together a list of specific ways that others can help—right now. Here's a list to get you started. Fill in every task that someone else can do to help you stay focused on taking care of yourself.

| Want to Help? Here's How... | Who/When |
| --- | --- |
| Call or e-mail updates to others in my "circle of care" | |
| Go with me to medical appointments and treatment sessions | |
| Participate in support groups | |
| Go shopping for me | |
| Cook my favorite foods—or things I can tolerate at this moment | |
| Provide childcare assistance, including driving kids to school and helping them with homework | |
| Clean the house | |
| Take care of pets | |
| Ensure that bills are paid on time | |
| Do laundry | |

## Talk to Your Family about Your Issues and Concerns

It's important to keep the lines of communication with your family as open as possible for the duration of your cancer treatment. Doing so will not only help you keep your emotions in check, but it will also help your family to understand where you are in the process of dealing with your disease.

Bottling up your feelings because you don't want to bring anyone else down is understandable at first, when your mind needs time to process everything that's happening to your body. But once you regain your footing, it's important to communicate as openly as possible with your caregiver, as well as your entire family. After all, their minds have been working overtime, too. Sharing your worries, fears, and concerns, as well as your hopes for the future, can be a positive bonding experience for all involved.

In an effort to pin down the sometimes swirling thoughts or ideas you might be experiencing, it might be helpful for you to keep a notebook of things you'd like to discuss with your family. Sometimes, just having a list can bring you both the comfort and confidence necessary to open up—especially if you tend to be a shy or private person.

The first time you have a discussion with family may be the most challenging. If you don't know where to start, use your list, or ask someone else to start talking about his or her feelings first. It won't be long before you're having one of the most real conversations you've ever shared as a group. Once you're done, celebrate this achievement for your family—moments like these will become anchors for all of you as you travel this new road together.

> We can talk for hours about prostate cancer with friends and acquaintances and expect our wives not only to listen ad nauseam, but also to agree with us at all times. We often become fixated with our problems…and the fear of our own mortality, while at the same time becoming oblivious to the needs of our spouse. We must remember that she not only has to deal with our mood swings, declining health, unusual diets, anxiety over PSA test results, and all the other issues relating to our disease—she must also face her own fears. Recognize her fears and the load she must carry. Ask yourself what you can do to make her life, now and after you're gone, a better life.
>
> —HARRY PINCHOT, A.K.A. "HELPLINE HARRY,"
> *participant, seven-year survivor,*
> *The Wellness Community - Valley/Ventura*

**Caregivers' Corner**

*Caregiving Basics*

Becoming a caregiver can be a wonderful spiritual and emotional calling, but it can also be a challenging labor of love. Here are some basic things you should do for your loved one:

- **Know the facts**.

    Learn as much as you can about the type of cancer your loved one has, including potential health issues and details regarding pain management

- **Make connections**.

    Your local hospital likely has a medical social worker who can help you learn more about caregiving, connecting you with a course or workshop on home care in your own community. Many visiting nurse services also provide home training for caregivers. The more you know, the more secure you'll feel

- **Learn how to manage pain and other side effects**.

    Don't wait for the pain to spike before you offer meds. Try to catch any pain as it starts, so the meds won't need to play "catch-up" to the pain. Always have sufficient medication on hand to help manage pain, nausea, and other side effects of cancer treatment

- **Keep germs away**.

    People with cancer have impaired immune systems and are more susceptible to illness as a result. Advise sick visitors to stay home. Keep and use alcohol-based instant hand sanitizer to minimize the spread of germs. When you need to, use latex or vinyl gloves

- **Respect privacy.**

    Don't just barge in on your loved one—and don't share personal details about his or her care or prognosis with anyone unless you have your loved one's permission

- **Don't do too much**.

    Don't assume your loved one needs you for everything. Ask if he or she needs help before giving it

- **Fight boredom.**

    Help alleviate the doldrums for both yourself and your loved one during treatments or home care. Bring movies, books, tapes, and games to share for times of bed rest

- **Honor quiet moments.**

    Soft music, aromatherapy (when tolerable), and warm baths offer much in the way of comfort—for both you and the patient

- **Listen**.

    Be your loved one's advocate when it's time for medical intervention

## Talking to Medical Professionals Effectively

As soon as your loved one was diagnosed, both of you became part of a new, bewildering world. Even if you've dealt with doctors, nurses, and hospitals previously, this time it's different.

As we often tell other caregivers at The Wellness Community, you play a vital role in dealing with medical professionals—both on your own behalf and in support of your loved one with cancer. You'll serve as the liaison between your loved one and his or her medical team, asking questions or raising concerns that are the patient's or your own. It's therefore quite important to develop a positive working relationship with the healthcare professionals who treat your loved one.

We suggest you build a "positive partnership" with your loved one's medical team by:

- **Asking questions**.

    Carry a notebook with you to every doctor's appointment and hospital stay. Jot down questions as they occur to you or your loved one. Keep a record of the patient's treatment experiences—both positive and negative. Be ready to talk to the doctor when he or she is available

- **Taking notes**.

    When the patient is seen by the doctor, keep notes on what was said to help manage your loved one's expectations relating to treatment, side effects, and general wellness. Keep details on whom or when to call in the event of an emergency

- **Relieving discomfort**.

    One of the most difficult moments in the caregiving process is when your loved one is in pain. Naturally, we want to do something—anything—as quickly as possible to help. But nurses and doctors have many patients in their care and may not always be able to respond immediately to your needs. Try not to be angry or upset with them once they do respond. Voice any concerns in quiet moments outside of the patient's room. Ask nurses what you can do to help your loved one to be more comfortable

- **Sharing hunches.**

    Often, as the person closest to the patient, you become aware of issues or changes before the medical team realizes they exist. If something doesn't seem right to you, there's a good chance it isn't. Be ready to share any hunches regarding your loved one's well-being. Remember, you are the patient's advocate—and in some cases, you may be your loved one's only voice

Most medical professionals respect caregivers who can express themselves as directly as possible, and are more than willing to work closely to offer the best care. But they don't always have time to have long discussions. So, take a deep breath, pull out your notes, and stay focused when discussing your loved one's care. Remember: you're all working together on the same team.

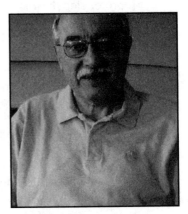

*I got through this terrible time with the help of my wife and my daughters, who were just wonderful. My wife and I are so thankful for our daughters' help.... My wife had her right cancerous kidney removed five days before my surgery. Without their help, I don't know how we would have managed.*

—Gilbert Ossandon,
*participant, The Wellness Community - Central New Jersey*

## Helping Children Understand

The shock of diagnosis was most definitely a challenge for you and your caregiver, but one of the toughest challenges for cancer patients with children in their lives is how and when to tell them about the cancer— even if the children in question are now adults. Let's face it, nothing in your role as a parent, grandparent, aunt, uncle, or family friend has prepared you for a challenge like this one.

However much you wish you could keep it "away from the children," cancer is an impossible secret to keep. Kids overhear phone conversations, feel their parents' anxiety, and imagine the worst possible scenarios when left to their own interpretations of what's going on. Adult children notice a growing distance in your relationship.

When a parent has cancer, the natural desire to protect the children usually backfires and makes things worse. If parents don't explain the situation with age-appropriate facts, their children may:

- Hear about a parent's cancer from someone else and have trouble trusting their parents afterward
- Think their parents are trying to conceal something and have trouble believing the truth when they are told
- Decide that whatever is happening is too terrible to be discussed, which can isolate them from the family
- Believe that they are to blame for the cancer because they have been angry with their mom or dad
- Worry that cancer is contagious, that everyone dies from it, or that they or the other parent will get it

Younger children need to be told that it isn't their fault and that cancer is not caused by their own negative behavior. Older children need to be given the chance to be part of the treatment and healing process, or they may feel resentful later on when you really need their support.

Children mirror the emotions of the adults around them. Therefore, how a child reacts depends very much on how well the parents or other close adults are dealing with their own feelings. School-aged children may find it hard to accept new expectations for help with younger siblings and household chores. Children of all ages fear the cancer will lead to the loss of the parent. Difficulty in discussing these issues may create distance in relationships that were once close—and this could lead to lifelong behavioral issues and emotional disorders.

## When to Seek Professional Help

Because children can't be shielded from all the stressful or challenging parts of life, it's important to teach them how to cope. Your cancer experience offers the learning opportunity of a lifetime—for all the members of your family, including yourself. Be the example; lead the way for your children as you embark on this new journey together.

Sometimes, unable to fully express their fears or feelings, some kids act out their emotional distress. Older kids might engage in risky behavior, using drugs, alcohol, or sex as a coping mechanism. The most important factor is how extreme the behavioral changes are and how long they have been going on. If you notice that things aren't right with your child, call the pediatrician, school guidance counselor, or medical social work/counseling staff at your treatment hospital. Let any or all of these professionals recommend a counselor who's experienced in working with children whose parents have a chronic illness. Many community organizations like The Wellness Community also offer special programs for kids who have a parent with cancer. With children, in particular, early intervention is the best prevention.

### Not an Easy Road
A recent study from the *Journal of Family Nursing (JFN)* shows that there can be a significant impact on your emotional, physical, and even financial health when you are dealing with a serious illness such as cancer. Nearly 62 percent of caregivers said their own health had suffered as a result of caring for a loved one, 70 percent said their families were just not working well together on a caregiving plan, and 46 percent said they had inadequate financial resources due to caregiving. In fact, nearly half of all personal bankruptcies in the U.S. today are due to medical expenses relating to serious illness.

## Seek Harmony

If your family was dysfunctional before the cancer, you really can't expect things to get better immediately after a diagnosis. However, sometimes it takes a life-threatening illness to jolt everyone back into reality. Try using the cancer as a catalyst for long-overdue family meetings or discussions. Tell your family that this cancer offers an opportunity for healing that extends far beyond your own physical body. Even if you're not directly involved in the family drama, tell the others that one of the best ways for them to help you is to heal their rifts and work through their issues so that you can all focus your energy on the challenging road ahead.

Moving your family from discord to harmony will add extra meaning to your cancer experience, making the journey even more worthwhile. You've got nothing to lose and everything to gain from trying.

## Connecting Family with Support Groups or Family Therapists

If, despite your best efforts, things still don't seem to be working for you or those close to you, it may be time to call in a professional team. Counseling can help people with cancer and their family members:

- Learn more effective ways to communicate about the illness
- Cope better with the normal feelings and reactions to cancer
- Address changes in roles and family routines that may result
- Relieve some of the emotional and physical side effects of the cancer and your treatments

There are twenty-three Wellness Communities that offer free support groups worldwide in addition to online support groups through The Virtual Wellness Community. *(See Appendix for resources and information on The Wellness Community and its locations.)*

You may also consider asking your healthcare team for a referral, or sharing your feelings with your minister, priest, or rabbi. You can determine which type of counselor might work best for your situation—the only bad choice is no choice.

## Joining Hands

The cancer journey is not one you should attempt to make alone. Involving others in decision-making and treatment, as well as general care, can ease the stress of dealing with your cancer—offering you added health benefits that could even extend your life.

Cancer is not a solitary disease; it's an illness that affects everyone who cares about you, as well. So, reach out and join hands to form a "circle of care." You'll be amazed—and blessed—by the results.

> **Patient Action Plan for Caregivers**
> Here are some ways you can take care of yourself when caring for a loved one:
> - **Don't try to be everything to everybody**.
>   You can't do it all—at least not right now. So forget about keeping your house, car, kids, job, pets, friendships, etc. in the manner to which they—and you—have been accustomed. Learn to say "no." You are in a crisis situation—and others should understand and work with you to keep things moving

- **Prioritize**.

  The main priority today is your loved one and his or her needs with respect to the cancer. The second priority is YOU and your immediate family. The third is your finances. Everything else will have to wait until you have time to deal with it

- **Delegate**.

  People want to help in a crisis. Let them! Delegate every responsibility you can. Remember that most people say "Is there anything I can do?" because they want to help but don't know what's needed. Show them your list; keep it in your notebook or near the phone at all times so that you can pencil in tasks to assign

- **Get or stay connected**.

  Join and participate in support groups for caregivers. If you can't get out to a group meeting, buddy up with another caregiver to share tips and experiences, or join an online support group, such as those provided by The Wellness Community. Also, if you have a lot of family members who want daily reports on your loved one's progress, consider starting an online group or blog to make daily postings. That way, you'll only need to capture experiences once, and others can chat amongst themselves as you conserve your energy to care for your loved one

- **Spend ten to thirty minutes a day on yourself**.

  Make sure you get a regular break by scheduling time for others to care for your loved one. Impossible, you say? Wrong. Ten minutes just looking out of a window at snow, birds, trees, or the ocean will help to keep you sane. Listen to music or go for a walk. Eat a chocolate bar or visit the gift shop. Watch a favorite television show or read a book in a place that's away from your loved one. The important thing is to reconnect with anything that makes you feel human again. You'll feel better and bring more positive energy back into the room—and you'll also have more to discuss than just the cancer. That's something your loved one will surely appreciate

## A Final Note for Caregivers

Taking time for you is not selfish. It's not a reflection on the quality of care you are providing for your loved one. Even if you're working hard to keep as normal a routine as possible, you still need time away in order to recharge your energies, as well as to avoid depression and/or burnout. Realize as early as possible that you can't do it all, and you will find that you can become a strengthened ally to the very person you most want to help through this difficult journey. Your loved one will benefit even more from being with you when you have a healthy balance of your own.

## Chapter 13

# Spirituality and Looking Inward

*We can spend lifetimes spinning stories about our boss being a jerk, what new car we want to buy next, how much money we're making, or how irritated we are with our mates and family, and about how right we are in all of those scenarios. What does all of that spinning do for us? We get dizzy and confused, never seeing the real truth, which is that we spend so much time looking outward, we fail to find the* 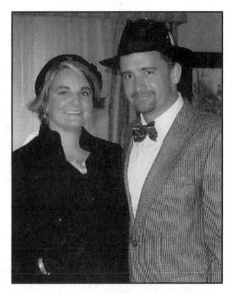 *real treasure only found by looking within. Whether we're already on some kind of inward journey or spiritual path, just beginning, or haven't sought the pathway just yet, cancer doesn't leave much choice but to look within. Cancer has led me to where my ego would never have wished to go because I was too afraid...and cancer has shown my soul exactly where I needed to be to find my depth and face my fears honestly.*

—Rebecca L. Tyrrell,
*caregiver participant,*
*The Wellness Community - Central Indiana*

**W**E ALL HAVE A spiritual dimension, whether or not we participate in a religious tradition. Each of us holds beliefs about life, its meaning, and its value. Feeling a sense of purpose and connection to a larger reality beyond the self can provide comfort while facing the challenges of cancer and may help you to put your situation into perspective. Prayer, meditation, and other spiritual practices can ease distress and be restorative, whether done in a religious institution or outdoors among nature.

If you or a loved one is diagnosed with cancer, you may find comfort in your spiritual beliefs—or you may question your faith. Many people ask "Why is this happening to me?" or "Why am I being punished?" In spite of current understandings about the multiple reasons why cancer occurs, the idea that the illness might be a punishment for some past sin or lack of faith continues to plague patients and their families. The best way to rid yourself of such irrational thoughts is to confront your "monsters" head-on. Work with a spiritual leader to find more effective ways of dealing with your grief, and, over time, your feelings of betrayal will dissipate. Know that you are not to blame for your cancer.

## Evaluating Your Life

Being diagnosed with a potentially life-threatening disease often forces people to take a reflective look at their lives. Some may conclude that they have not accomplished enough, loved enough, or contributed enough to the world. Others may feel satisfied with where they are and what they have accomplished. The crisis of cancer can serve to help people gain insights into their beliefs and experiences and, thereby, promote personal growth.

People with cancer who have a religious affiliation may find it useful to meet with a representative of their faith, such as a minister, priest, rabbi, or other clerical person, or a respected member of the religious community. This "religious guide" may be able to help you search for answers to difficult questions of faith that often arise. It may be reassuring to remember that having doubts or being angry is a normal response to facing cancer and its resulting changes.

You may be able to meet with a pastoral counselor in the hospital or through a community-based counseling agency. Because not everyone is experienced in the emotional and spiritual issues you might face when dealing with cancer, seek out someone else if the person you contact doesn't meet your needs. Hospice programs also provide spiritual counseling. These services are usually available to the community free of charge.

Members of religious and spiritual communities may also provide practical help, such as assistance with transportation, meals, visitation services, and emotional support.

## The Power of Faith and Prayer

If prayer has helped you deal with other troubles, it will probably be comforting now and may help you feel less alone. Prayer and scientifically tested cancer treatments can coexist, and there's some evidence to suggest that spiritual practices, such as prayer, may assist in medical treatment, for example, by reducing hospital stays and increasing quality of life.

Medical professionals are also beginning to make a stronger connection between spirituality and medical treatment. Andrew Weil, M.D., author and founder of the Center for Integrative Medicine, writes: "It's obvious to me that grief and depression impair resistance and health in general, so I would not be surprised to learn that mental and spiritual imbalances make people more susceptible to cancer. Working to improve mental/spiritual health...cannot fail to bolster defenses against all kinds of disease, including cancer" (Weil).

Because having a sense of life's meaning beyond the self can help improve your quality of life and provide inner peace, strengthen your spirit in whatever ways work best for you. Some possible activities that may be helpful are prayer, meditation, reading spiritual writings, attending religious services, helping others, doing yoga, surrounding yourself with nature, listening to music, and spending time with loved ones.

> *I feel truly blessed. [Cancer] was my wake-up call. I cannot imagine the wonderful friends and love I have received over the past years would have been a part of my life without having had cancer.*
>
> —JUDITH OPAHL,
> *former participant and current executive director,*
> *The Wellness Community - South Bay Cities*

## Affirmation: Saying Is Believing

A powerful tool for framing a positive outcome, affirmation is the art of creating positive thoughts that help you to see beyond your situation and act "as if." These thoughts are useful in helping you to maintain a strong sense of control over your illness, but they can also serve as the seeds of self-fulfilling prophecy.

Because there's great benefit in repetition, affirmations work best when used daily and when strategically placed throughout your home or office so that you are reminded of them often. You may use some affirmations from a book or create your own using this list as a starting point:

> *I continue to be a healthy person with a joyous life.*
> *I lovingly care for myself every step of the way.*
> *I embrace every opportunity for healing that I encounter along my path.*
> *My spirit looks exactly the same, regardless of changes in my body.*
> *I am safe and whole and open to new possibilities in my life.*
> *I continue to participate fully in as many activities as I choose.*
> *Everything is happening for my highest good.*
> *I am the creator of my own health and happiness.*
> *I am in complete control of all of my options and will make all the right decisions regarding my treatment and care.*
> *I am truly grateful for all that I have and all that I am.*

## Connecting with Your Personal Source of Happiness

Whether or not you are faith-based and pray regularly, there's always another way to express your deepest hopes, fears, and feelings—safely and creatively. You can draw, paint, or write in a journal. Or perhaps you can express yourself with music or quiet walks in the park.

However you choose to connect with your powerful inner soul, if you do so with hope and optimism about the future, whatever it may hold, you will be a much happier—and healthier—human being. And that's exactly what it will take to help fight your cancer and increase your potential for long-term survival.

*When people comment about the fact that I am a walking miracle, I respond, 'You are right!' I'm still amazed that I'm alive. My faith is stronger, and my life has changed. After looking death in the face and battling for my life four times, I don't sweat the small stuff . . . and yearn to let family and friends all over the world know that their compassion, words of encouragement, cleaning the house, financial assistance, meals, and rides to the doctor appointments mean more than they can ever imagine. While each of us is different as we journey through treatment, know that we need your prayers and understanding. It's a job too big for any one person, regardless of the amount of faith and love. It's never ending.*

—SHERRY B. WILLIAMS,
*participant, The Wellness Community - Central Arizona*

**Patient Action Plan**
- **To help you deal with negative emotions, look inward—or reach outward.**
  Connect with what resonates or inspires you on a spiritual level
- **Evaluate the quality of your life.**
  Focus your energy on the good that you have shared with others, as this kind of sharing is what connects you with the healing love of others
- **Practice the power of prayer.**
  Even if it's just allowing others to pray for you
- **Learn to use affirmations in your daily life.**
  One way to do that is to write and post healing quotations or thoughts around the house or office—in places where you will see them every day

# Part Four

# Moving from Patient Active to Life Active

## Chapter 14

# Reaching Out
## Networking and Connecting with Resources

*It's hard to explain to people who have no experience with cancer that [The Wellness Community] is a happy place, and that I get 200 percent back for my time put in. If you can help one person, it's worth it. The people who work at our TWC are all family to me, and it's so wonderful to come to a place where you're needed, respected, and loved. The hope on participants' faces is the icing on the cake.*

—CAROL LYSTAD,
*participant/volunteer,*
*The Wellness Community - Southwest Florida*

IMAGINE YOURSELF SITTING IN a room with ten other people who have cancer. Just last week, your doctor, as well as other people in her waiting room, suggested that you attend such a gathering. So, here you are—a new member of a cancer support group, which begins with the professional facilitator asking you if you would like to share anything about your cancer experience. Perhaps you might share what type of cancer you have, when you were diagnosed, and what treatments you are going through. You may also choose to share what you are feeling and how cancer has impacted your life. In the moment before you answer, you pause and reflect: "Why am I here? Will participating in a support group *really* help me—and if so, how?"

For the last twenty-five years, there's been extensive research on the positive effects of support groups as a method of coping with cancer, improving quality of life, and in some studies even increasing survival. Research has shown that support groups help reduce the three most significant stressors associated with cancer: unwanted aloneness, loss of control, and loss of hope.

For example, in controlled studies at Stanford University and the University of California, Los Angeles, psychological distress and pain were significantly reduced while quality of life significantly improved in women who participated in breast cancer support groups (1). Some studies have even shown increased survival as a result of support group participation (2). More recently, in a replication of previous research, Pamela J. Goodwin, M.D., and her colleagues found that, although women in professionally facilitated support groups did not survive longer, they experienced significant quality of life improvements—they were less distressed and suffered less pain (Goodwin et al.)

Community-based, rather than hospital- or university-based, cancer support programs also lend further evidence that support groups can be beneficial (4). In non-randomized studies of community-based cancer support programs, results have shown that participants generally rate their experiences as positive and beneficial (McLean; Taylor et al.; Glajchen & Moul; Gray et al.; Helgeson et al.).

In a study done at The Wellness Community with Stanford University, findings suggest that support groups in the community that encourage preparing for the worst while hoping for the best may reduce cancer patients' overall distress (Taylor et al.; Glajchen & Moul; McLean; Taylor et al.; Glajchen & Moul; Gray et al.; Helgeson et al.). Although TWC is awaiting final outcomes from this study, the women in the community-based support groups benefited at about the same rate as those women who participated in the more formal Stanford University study, in terms of reduced depression and trauma symptoms, as well as improved social support, self-efficacy, and post-traumatic-growth. This is encouraging news for people participating in professionally facilitated, community-based cancer support groups—especially at TWC, with its wide geographic reach.

*It was nearly a year ago that I first came to The Wellness Community. Newly diagnosed with cancer of unknown primary, I stood at the door, looking for hope. A light rain was falling, and I was having difficulty finding the strength to open the door and enter. I stood on the steps crying, thinking how unfair this all was, and that once I entered, I would truly admit that I had cancer. As I tried to compose myself, I heard a voice from inside. The voice said, 'I don't know why* 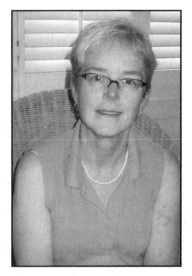 *you're crying, but I can't help you until you step inside.' The door opened, and I became a participant [that day].*

—BETH BOOKER,
*participant, The Wellness Community - East Tennessee*

## The Wellness Community Model

The Wellness Community provides a fertile environment to translate recent scientific discoveries in the field of psychosocial oncology directly into psychosocial support programs that improve the day-to-day lives of people fighting for recovery from cancer. Since 1996, TWC has been actively engaged in community-initiated research collaborations with several academic research partners, including Stanford University, the University of California at San Francisco, and other educational institutions. Founded in 1982, TWC reached more than 200,000 people with cancer and their loved ones in the past year through visits to our centers, visits to our Virtual Wellness Community, and through the distribution of our award-winning patient education materials. 30,000 people with cancer make about 200,000 visits to TWC's twenty-three national centers each year, attending support groups and educational and wellness programs, including physician lectures, meditation, and exercise and nutrition workshops—all free of charge. Our support groups are led by licensed psychotherapists specially trained in TWC's unique program methodology.

The program is based upon founder Dr. Harold Benjamin's Patient Active Concept: People with cancer who participate in their fight for recovery, along with their physician and healthcare team, will not only improve their quality of life, but may enhance the possibility of recovery. This approach combines the will of the patient with the skill of the physician during cancer treatment and beyond.

TWC's Patient Active program has been described as an empowerment model where people are:

- Making active choices in their recovery
- Making changes in their lives that they think are important
- Partnering with their physicians
- Accessing resources
- Developing new attitudes toward the illness

Moreover, the program emphasizes reducing the three most significant psychosocial stressors faced by people with cancer—unwanted aloneness, loss of control, and loss of hope. It's these aspects of The Wellness Community model that are important new discoveries in improving quality of life for people with cancer and their loved ones.

> *I walked in and immediately felt comfort. First, the physical environment was so consoling to my spirit—it just felt like home. And then, the 'walking, talking' survivors with beautiful, welcoming smiles on their faces made me so relieved that there were other 'Warrior Women' who have battled the war on this disease—and are winning!*

—KRYSTI HUGHETT,
*participant, The Wellness Community - Central Indiana*

## The Internet and Cancer Support

Today, it's hard to imagine what life would be like without e-mail and access to the Internet. We take it for granted. But the idea that you could receive cancer support and information via the Internet that's just as helpful as the support or information you receive in a face-to-face support group or workshop is still revolutionary. The technology that enables those people with cancer who are too ill or live too far from support services to receive these services via the Internet allows access for millions more people dealing with cancer. This revolution is taking place and, more recently, there's research to support its value.

> ## A Growing Trend
> To capture the immensity of this health-information revolution, consider these facts:
> - Research from a PEW Poll (November 2006) found that 80 percent of all those who currently use the Internet have looked for health information on the Web. This represents 113 million adults (McLean; Taylor et al.; Glajchen & Moul; Gray et al.; Helgeson et al.)
> - The PEW Foundation released a report in 2003 stating that 25.2 million Americans have contacted a support group for help
> - In 2004, 36 million have become members of a support group for help
> - In 2006, 58 percent of those who sought health information reported that the information they received influenced their treatment decisions

## Do Online Support Groups Really Help?

Have you ever wondered whether these Internet-based support groups actually help? An important 2003 study found that women with breast cancer who participated in professionally facilitated online support groups scheduled in "real time" (modeled after The Wellness Community's face-to-face support groups) experienced significant decreases in depression and negative reactions to pain, as well as significant increases in zest for life and spirituality (Cordova et al.). Another study offering professionally moderated support groups that were not in "real time" and included semi-structured topics also showed significant decreases in depression, perceived stress, and cancer-related trauma (Lieberman et al.).

In a comparison of face-to-face support groups to Online Support Groups (OSGs), both offered through TWC for women with breast cancer, participants derived similar support and access to information in both groups. Similarly, the facilitators in both settings played nearly identical roles helping participants express emotions, reframe experiences, and learn from each other (Winzelberg et al.). So, while there's a need for continuing research, it appears that those participating in on-line support groups are receiving similar benefits to those participating in face-to-face groups. These results are promising in that many more people with cancer can now be served.

In February 2002, as a result of these findings, TWC launched The Virtual Wellness Community (TVWC) at www.thewellnesscommunity.org. The Web site mirrors a physical Wellness Community with free, professionally moderated support groups. It hosts physician lectures, mind-body programs, and other services for people affected by cancer. The brick-and-mortar Wellness Communities create home-like settings for their participants; The Virtual Wellness Community does the same. There's a mind-body room, library, and kitchen filled with nutrition information—and the best part is, it's always open.

> **Key Features . . . with Lots of Benefits**
> Here are the main features of online support groups in TWC's Virtual Wellness Community:
> - Meet weekly at a scheduled time for ninety minutes. Include no more than eight participants
> - Facilitated by licensed professionals trained in The Wellness Community's model
> - Offer downloadable relaxation/meditation sessions, as well as sessions with speakers of note

Currently, there are free online support groups at The Virtual Wellness Community and at other Web sites for people with a variety of diagnoses, including breast, prostate, lung, ovarian, pancreatic, and colorectal cancers, and lymphoma. These sites are also useful to caregiver groups. TWC also offers similar program services in Spanish (espanol.thewellnesscommunity.org). TVWC has received more than 9 million hits since its introduction and more than 200,000 unique visitors.

While there are a multitude of places on the Internet to find information and engage in discussion with other survivors, it's important to be careful about what information you may be receiving. For online support groups or chat rooms, ask if the sessions are professionally facilitated or moderated. This can help to create a safe environment that's a good place to share information and feelings (Benjamin).

*While my cancer is a long-standing problem, I have been involved with The Wellness Community for only a few months. I have been aware of support groups for cancer patients but seemed unable to find one that felt my situation was completely compatible with other participants' concerns—or was unable to find one that was accessible. At the last group meeting before this* 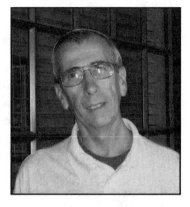 *writing, I decided to put the 'big underlying issue' for me on the table.... It is an indication that I feel comfortable with the process and other participants. TWC became an important lifeline for me after a few sessions.*

—LOUIS P. DEVOE,
*participant, The Wellness Community - Foothills*

## Benefits of a Virtual Wellness Community Support Group

As we discussed earlier in this chapter, research indicates that there are three significant psychosocial stressors among people who have cancer: loss of hope, feelings of unwanted aloneness, and loss of control. Each of these negative emotions can cause a great deal of stress that could suppress your immune system—your body's first line of defense against cancer. In your support group, you'll explore new ways to deal with the stressors associated with cancer and with life in general.

The Virtual Wellness Community Online Support Group program can help you:

- **Restore feelings of hope.**
  At TVWC, you'll meet and hear about many people who've survived cancer. The American Cancer Society says that there are more than ten million cancer survivors in the United States—for many of whom cancer is only a memory. In your support group, you'll find that there's always hope, even if what you are hoping for changes. Hope can give you a sense that life's worth living and

there's a reason to go on, even if you're in the final stages of the disease

- **Reduce feelings of unwanted aloneness.**

  Our support groups at TWC create opportunities to address the unwanted aloneness brought about by a cancer diagnosis by providing a safe, caring community of support. Learning that you're not alone by connecting with others who have had or are facing cancer can help you gain insight and understanding into your own perceptions and concerns about cancer, its treatment, and its impact upon your life. No matter how loved and supported by family and friends you may feel, it's normal to feel as if no one really understands unless he has been through it himself—hence, the value of being in an online or in-person support group

- **Regain a sense of control.**

  Participating in any TWC support group can also empower you to regain and maintain as much control of your life as is desirable. For example, when people in your group share information, life experiences, and concerns with each other, together they can explore issues of loss of control and whether they are giving up more control in their lives than is desirable or necessary. As a result of these group discussions, you can decide whether taking steps to address your situation better will help you feel more in control and, thereby, improve your quality of life

> **Accessibility Matters Most**
> The Wellness Community's online support groups offer the additional benefit of accessing services no matter where you are. Issues such as lack of programs in your area, travel time, or feeling too ill to leave your home are no longer obstacles in obtaining support services. We're always here for you!

## Support Group Guidelines

The Wellness Community weekly support groups—both online and face-to-face—are for people involved in the day-to-day fight for recovery from cancer. Once you or your significant other are without symptoms, or "cancer-free," for approximately eighteen months, you'll be expected to leave your weekly group. You're then welcome to take advantage of all of the other valuable resources in The Virtual Wellness Community.

The following are some important guidelines that we have learned help make face-to-face and online support groups a productive experience for as many people as possible:

- Make a commitment to attend group every week you're able. We recognize that there will be situations related to your treatment and personal life that may interfere with coming to group. Countless participants have shared that regular attendance improves the overall group experience. However, if you miss three meetings in a row without notifying the group, we'll have to assume you have dropped out
- If you're unable to attend a group meeting, please leave a message in the Discussion Board for those in online support groups, or for those in face-to-face support groups, contact your facilitator or a fellow participant via e-mail or phone. If possible, leave an explanation of why you're missing the group; because your group often becomes like an extended "family," members will be concerned when you're absent. Your fellow group members will want to know if your absence is due to a medically related problem or to something wonderful they can celebrate for you instead
- Arrive on time for the group. If you come late or miss group frequently, this may be an indication that group support isn't the right approach for you. Feel free to discuss this issue with your group, especially if you're not sure whether group is right for you
- Stay for the entire one-and-a-half-hour session. If for any reason you need to leave early, let the group know at the beginning of the meeting
- If you are in an online support group, you will be able to access The Virtual Wellness Community online support groups from anywhere, including the comfort of your own home, but it's important that you're in an environment that's as free of distraction as possible
- If you think you may want to change to a different group, you should discuss it with the group. If there's a practical reason for change, such as a new job with different hours or a shift in treatment schedules, the appropriate change can be made

The demand for participation in online support groups may be high and, therefore, may postpone a switch to another group. You should also be aware that, periodically, interns or staff-in-training may join your group.

By following these guidelines, not only will you make your support group experience more successful, you'll also receive the best support possible.

## Being "New" to a Support Group

When you're new to a support group, you may feel anxiety about what to do or how to act. After a very short time, though, you'll probably feel like "one of the family." In general, people are often surprised at how comfortable they feel, even if they never saw themselves before as a "support group" kind of person.

We suggest that you come to group for at least three or four weeks before deciding it's not right for you. If, after attending several sessions, you still feel that the group doesn't meet your needs, you should feel comfortable leaving the group. It's always best to be open with your group members about your concerns, as they might be able to help you figure out what's best for you.

We recognize that support groups aren't for everyone. Remember, there are a variety of ways to be Patient Active, both at TWC and elsewhere. You're always welcome to use our comprehensive TWC programs online or at any of our centers in any way that you believe best supports your fight for recovery.

## Sharing and Caring

People who are willing to share their experiences, thoughts, and feelings tend to receive more benefit from being in a group than those who don't. This type of sharing of oneself is an important way to build feelings of closeness and camaraderie. The Wellness Community should be the one place where you don't have to pretend, hold back, or feel you have to protect others from your fears and anxieties.

## The Facilitator's Role

At The Wellness Community, the unique role of the professional facilitator is a critical factor that sets our support groups apart from any other. Your TWC group facilitator is trained to help the group establish the framework of the meeting and provide a safe, compassionate environment for people to connect with one another in productive and meaningful ways. Your facilitator will share in the discussions, as appropriate, and include some of his or her personal views, feelings, and concerns. TWC group facilitators are experienced at understanding how groups work effectively, as well as in the aims and goals of TWC, but you're far more knowledgeable about navigating cancer and the effect it has had on your life. It's the expertise of your personal experience that you bring to share with group as a whole. In doing so, you not only help yourself, but you also discover how much you can help others.

As a participant, you're the real expert. You know more about your life and what to do with it than anyone else in the world. Every decision you make about your life will be the right one for you. The facilitator and your group members are there to *help you* look at the issues, ask the hard questions, and make the difficult decisions—not to make them for you.

It's best that you refrain from asking your facilitator to talk with you privately to discuss a problem that you think you wouldn't feel comfortable talking about within the group. Most likely, your facilitator will suggest that it's your responsibility to bring that information back to the group, because we believe you'll gain much more by bringing it in yourself, including a positive feeling of having taken control of that piece of your life. Also, by bringing your concerns and problems to group, even if it's about the group itself, you can receive benefit from the feedback of others who have gone through similar situations or have similar or dissimilar points of view.

Finally, The Virtual Wellness Community's online support groups are educational and informational and are not intended as psychotherapy. The facilitator's role is to help keep the group focused and help participants interact more fully with each other. Although no doctor-patient relationship is intended or implied, you should know that we've done our very best to ensure that your online experience is the most helpful, positive, and encouraging one it can be.

**Patient Action Plan**
- **Become more interested in the lives of your group members.**

    The more interested you are in them, the more interested they'll be in you. This unique friendship is built on shared experiences and can serve as an antidote to unwanted aloneness. Even if you don't feel like it, consider taking a chance to share your thoughts and concerns to see if it's helpful

- **Take an active part in group discussions by asking questions and giving feedback.**

    This enhances how you can relate more meaningfully with others, thereby strengthening the value—both personal and for the group—of the time you spend together

- **Get to know the members of your group as individuals through the Discussion Board, telephone calls, e-mails, or in any other mutually agreeable way.**

    Let other members of the group know whether you want to be contacted. Discuss your limits. Don't expect others to guess them

- **Participate actively in your group, but at your own pace.**

    Warming up to new people is easier for some people than for others. If simply getting online and listening to others works for you, then start with that, and get comfortable with being in a group experience

## Chapter 15

# Wellness Inside and Out
## Nutrition and Exercise*

**\*Adapted from material by Carolyn Katzin**

*Nutrition classes boost my physical well-being and teach me how to cook healthy meals. [At The Wellness Community], social programs had potluck dinners focused on holidays like Mardi Gras, and Halloween. These were fun and enjoyable!*

—LORRAINE TWARDOWKSI,
*participant,*
*The Wellness Community -*
*Delaware*

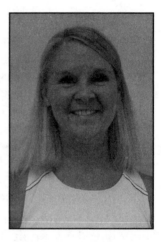

GOOD DIET IS ESPECIALLY important during any illness because the body requires nutrients both to fight the disease and to heal from the disease and treatments. However, maintaining healthy eating habits is often difficult for people with cancer. Many patients don't feel like eating for a variety of reasons, such as the side effects of the treatments; emotional factors, including depression and anxiety; or the chemical changes that cancer itself can cause. Nutritional services may be available and helpful if you're having trouble eating and maintaining your weight.

## Treatment-Related Nutritional Concerns

Chemotherapy, radiation, surgery, and immunotherapy are powerful tools designed to kill cancer cells, but they can also affect normal, healthy cells and cause conditions that may result in nutritional problems.

Surgery may lessen the ability of the mouth, throat, and stomach to work properly, making these areas sore and slowing digestion. Radiation therapy can cause mucositis, diarrhea, nausea, and vomiting, and can affect the body's ability to absorb nutrients. The effects of chemotherapy on nutrition will depend on the type of drug, dosage, duration of treatment, rates of excretion, and other individual factors. Chemotherapy can cause diarrhea, nausea and vomiting, loss of appetite, changes in the way food tastes and smells, a sore mouth and/or throat, and constipation.

There are many nutritional products that can be used to supplement reduced food intake, such as high-calorie and/or high-protein liquid preparations. These products can be used along with regular meals, in-between meals, or instead of meals. In addition, drinking protein-fortified beverages or adding one-quarter to one-third cup of non-fat dry milk to one cup of fluid milk can increase protein and calories.

Some patients have lactose intolerance, or difficulty in digesting or absorbing the milk sugar called lactose, following chemotherapy or abdominal radiation. Symptoms may include bloating, cramping, or gas several hours after eating milk products. Adding an enzyme (available in tablets or liquid drops) to break down the lactose or using lactose-reduced dairy products may make it possible to use milk and other dairy products, which are an excellent source of calories and protein.

> **The American Cancer Society's Nutrition Guidelines**
> The National Cancer Institute estimates that at least 35 percent of all cancers are linked to diet. For women, this is as high as *one half* of all cancers. Good nutrition is vital for a healthy immune system, which protects us from and provides resistance to cancer. Here's a summary of the American Cancer Society's guidelines for individual choices:
>
> **Eat a Variety of Healthful Foods, with an Emphasis on Plant Sources**:
> - Eat five or more servings of a variety of vegetables and fruits each day
> - Choose whole grains in preference to processed (refined) grains and sugars

- Limit consumption of red meats, especially those processed and high in fat
- Choose foods that help maintain a healthy weight

**Adopt a Physically Active Lifestyle**:
- Adults: Engage in at least moderate activity for thirty minutes or more on five or more days of the week; forty-five minutes or more of moderate to vigorous activity on five or more days per week may further enhance reductions in the risk of colon cancer
- Children and adolescents: Engage in at least sixty minutes per day of moderate to vigorous physical activity at least five days per week

**Maintain a Healthy Weight throughout Life**:
- Balance caloric intake with physical activity
- Lose weight if currently overweight or obese
- If you drink alcoholic beverages, limit consumption

## Dietary Guidelines throughout the Treatment Cycle

If you've been diagnosed with cancer, nutrition is one of the most important things for you to consider as part of your whole treatment regimen. Having a healthy diet can make a big difference in the success of your treatment. A simple rule of thumb is to maintain a steady body weight throughout treatment as much as possible. This means neither gaining nor losing too much weight (fluctuations of more than, say, five pounds per week for an average-sized adult). Balance your intake with physical activity to your own individual capacity.

*Before Treatment*:

*Surgery*: Eat a low-fat (less than 25 percent of calories), high-protein (8–10 oz. lean meat, fish, chicken, or turkey) diet the day before surgery. Supplement with a broad spectrum multi-vitamin and mineral with 100 percent recommended dietary allowances (RDA). Additionally, 500 mg vitamin C with bioflavonoid every eight hours may be beneficial to healing. Stop supplements of vitamin E, vitamin K, evening primrose, borage, or fish oils one week before surgery, as these can cause thinning of the blood.

*Radiation*: No special diet.

*Chemo*: Eat a low-fat, high-carbohydrate diet the day before chemotherapy. No supplements on day of treatment.

## During Treatment:

*Surgery*: As per surgeon's protocol.

*Radiation*: Extra carbohydrate calories for energy.

*Chemo*: Avoid eating your favorite foods within twenty-four hours of treatment to avoid negative associations with them at a later time. Eat a low-fat (less than 3 tablespoons or 40 grams fat/oil per day), high-carbohydrate (mainly complex carbohydrate or starch from grains, fruits, and vegetables) diet with small quantities of good-quality protein. White-meat chicken, fish, and eggs are easy to digest. Protein powder-based smoothies are also good. Avoid more than RDA amounts of antioxidant supplements.

## After Treatment:

*Surgery*: High-protein diet (8–10 oz. lean meat, poultry, fish, or 2–3 eggs). Regular supplements as above. Antioxidant supplement including 400 IU vitamin E and 1,000 mg vitamin C per day.

*Radiation*: High-protein and energy diet. Lactose-free and relatively low in simple sugars (sucrose and honey) to avoid intestinal discomfort.

*Chemo*: Small, frequent meals of easy-to-digest foods such as fish, chicken, rice, baked potato, banana, or applesauce. Stimulate appetite with ginger ale. If weight drops rapidly, add a smoothie and/or meal replacement type products. Avoid lactose, as above.

> **Nutrition and Chemotherapy:**
> - Drink plenty of fluids (at least two liters total), with most of it coming from clear liquids such as water, apple juice, and clear broths—and/or eat Jell-O®. Avoid caffeine-containing liquids such as tea, coffee, and colas, as these are dehydrating
> - Eat small quantities of food rather than large meals for easier digestion
> - Eat crackers, Melba toast, pasta, and baked potato if you feel nauseated
> - Use the concept of the Expedient Diet, and make up for eating less healthily when you have more strength
> - Eat avocado often, as it is an excellent source of calories, essential fatty acids, potassium, and glutathione, unless you are contraindicated (if on procarbazine or other medication requiring a low-tyramine diet)

| Drug-Specific Nutritional Advice | |
|---|---|
| Asparaginase, Elspar | Drink extra fluids. Consume extra calories. |
| Bleomycin, Blenoxane | Bland foods. |
| Busulfan, Myleran | Drink extra fluids. Eat foods rich in B vitamins. |
| Carmustine, BiCNU | Bland foods, avocado. |
| Chlorambucil, Leukeran | Drink extra fluids. Bland foods, avocado. |
| Cisplatin and carboplatin | Avoid purine-rich foods (liver, caviar, sardines, anchovies). Eat plenty of magnesium, potassium, and zinc-rich foods (whole grains and nuts). Drink extra fluids. |
| Cladribine, 2-CdA, Leustatin | No special diet. |
| Cyclophosphamide, Cytoxan | Drink extra fluids. Don't cut back on salt or sodium-containing foods. Avoid alcohol. Eat bland and low-fat foods. |
| Cytarabine, Ara-C, Cytosar-U | Drink extra fluids. Bland foods, avocado. |
| Dacarbazine, DITC-Dome | Drink extra fluids. Bland foods, avocado. |
| Daunorubicin, Cerubidine | Drink extra fluids. Eat foods rich in B vitamins, particularly riboflavin (milk, lean meat, egg yolks, wheat germ). |
| Doxorubicin, Adriamycin | Drink extra fluids. Eat foods rich in B vitamins, particularly riboflavin (see above). |
| Etoposide, VePesid, VP-16 | Bland foods, avocado. |
| 5-Fluorouracil, Adrucil | Drink extra fluids. Eat foods rich in B vitamins. |
| Fludarabine, Fludara-IV | Drink extra fluids. |
| Hydroxyurea, Hydrea | Drink extra fluids. |
| Idarubicin, Idamycin | Drink extra fluids. |
| Ifosfamide, Ifex | Drink extra fluids. |
| Lomustine, CeeNU | Bland foods, avocado. |
| Mechlorethamine, Mustargen | Drink extra fluids. Restrict simple sugars. |
| Melphalan, Alkeran | Drink extra fluids. |
| Mercaptopurine, Purinethol | Drink extra fluids. Avoid alcohol. Avoid foods rich in purines (anchovies, kidneys, liver, meat extracts, sardines, beans, and lentils). Eat foods rich in B vitamins, like wheat germ. |

| Methotrexate, Mexate | Drink extra fluids. Avoid alcohol. Bland diet. Eat foods that produce an alkaline urine to assist excretion (almonds, milk, fruits and vegetables except cranberries, plums, corn, and lentils). |
|---|---|
| Mitomycin, Mutamycin | Drink extra fluids. Bland diet, avocado. Eat foods rich in folate (green, leafy vegetables, citrus fruits) and foods rich in calcium (dairy foods and broccoli). |
| Mitoxantrone, Novantrone | Drink extra fluids. (should have discolored urine) |
| Pentostatin, Nipent | Bland foods, avocado. |
| Procarbazine, Matulane | Avoid tyramine-containing foods (aged cheeses, yogurt, raisins, eggplant, canned figs, salami, sour cream, avocados, bananas, soy sauce, lima beans, tenderized meats, etc. Ask for a list from doctor). Maintain tyramine-free diet for fourteen days after treatment ceases. No alcohol. |
| Tamoxifen, Nolvadex | Avoid high-fat foods. Exercise regularly to minimize possible weight-gain side effect. Eat foods rich in calcium and magnesium (dairy foods, broccoli, nuts, and seeds). |
| Taxol | Drink extra fluids. |
| 6-Thioguanine, Tabloid | High-fiber diet. |
| Vinblastine, Velban | Drink extra fluids. |
| Vincristine, Oncovin | Drink extra fluids. Bland diet, avocado. |
| **New Anti-Cancer Agents** | |
| Interferon (recombinant Intron, Roferon) | Drink extra fluids. Bland diet, avocado. |
| Other cytokines | Eat plenty of protein. |
| **Drugs Used with Chemotherapy** | |
| Dexamethasone, Decadron | Low-salt, high-potassium diet (avocado, bananas, citrus fruits, most vegetables). Adequate chromium in diet (whole grains and brewer's yeast). |
| Prednisone, Deltasone | Low-sugar diet. No alcohol. |
| Meticorten, Orasone | Low-salt, high-potassium diet. No alcohol. Adequate chromium in diet (see above). |
| Mesna, Mesnex | Plenty of fluids. |

If your oncologist is using combinations of medications, modify the advice so that you retain the most important parts. Remember to speak with your doctor about nutrition. Ask for a dietary consult with a registered dietitian or certified nutrition specialist.

Here's an example of dietary advice for a combination regimen: "Avoid fatty foods. Eat small quantities of bland flavors. Avoid alcohol, highly spiced foods, or very acidic foods (cranberries, pineapple, lemons, etc.). Focus on vegetables, lean meats moistened in liquids, in stews or in soups, and on whole grain cereals. Many chemotherapy regimens affect your blood cell count. If not contraindicated, a hematinic (blood-building) supplement may be recommended. Check with your oncologist."

*Six years ago, I began to have pain in my lower back, and a CT scan showed a three-centimeter tumor on my kidney. After three opinions, we chose to do chemo (VCP) for six weeks and then Rituxan. The Rituxan was easily tolerated, and, within eight months, all visible tumors had gone. To date, I still get nodes that appear and disappear on their own. I know I have cancer, but I feel that by being fit and eating well, my cancer remains under control.*

—MATTHEW ACCARDO,
*participant, The Wellness Community -
South Bay Cities*

## Radiation Treatment and Nutrition

Radiation may affect your taste buds; food may now taste bitter, or you may have a metallic taste in your mouth. Try marinating meats for better flavor. Cold foods may be more palatable than hot. Use herbs such as thyme, tarragon, mint, or basil for added flavor. Try adding sauces such as applesauce, yogurt dressings, or salad dressings to make food easier to chew. Snack on whey or soy protein powder milk shakes. Ensure® or other canned elemental diets are also useful standbys; look for the newer versions suitable for radiation enteritis or other chronic diarrhea situations (e.g. Boost® or Resolve®). For maximum effects, radiation treatment should not be combined with high-dose supplements of antioxidants (beta carotene, vitamins C and E, or glutathione). The amounts found in a normal mixed diet will not interfere with treatment.

To counteract gastrointestinal problems, take additional B complex vitamins as nine tablets of brewer's yeast per day or in a supplement. You can also try four fluid ounces of aloe vera juice as a soothing drink. Avoid milk and milk products, as lactose intolerance may develop. Yogurt made from a live culture may be tolerated well. Use lactose-free milk or whey products to minimize discomfort with dairy products; Ensure and similar meal replacement drinks are lactose-free.

**Other Nutritional Helpers:**
- **Garlic**
  Allicin (allythio sulfinic allyl ester) is a weak anticancer agent found in garlic. Recognized as early as 1550 B.C. as a treatment for cancer
- **Pycnogenol**
  This powerful antioxidant is found in grape seeds and from an extract of pine trees. Anyone with alcohol-related liver damage should not take this or megadoses of beta-carotene for the same reasons
- **Milk Thistle (Silymarin)**
  This herb may assist in detoxification and general support of the liver detoxification enzyme systems. Useful after chemotherapy
- **Coenzyme Q10**
  This is another antioxidant that can be beneficial during treatment. Take 50–150 mg per day, or as directed by your nutrition professional
- **Green Papaya and Pineapple**
  Many tropical fruits contain natural enzymes that may be beneficial preventively and during treatment
- **Green Tea**
  Contains protective botanical factors. Drink some daily

## Natural Energy Drinks

Many treatments for cancer can leave you feeling depleted of energy. Not only that, but food may also taste bland and uninteresting. Here are some recipes to stimulate your appetite and lift your spirits in a natural way. A garnish of fresh fruit or mint adds appeal.

### Fruit Shake

*1 cup plain low-fat yogurt*
*1 ripe banana*
*A few drops vanilla extract*

*1 teaspoon honey*
*1 teaspoon coconut (optional)*

Blend a few ice cubes for a few minutes in a blender, then add the ingredients, and blend until smooth. The banana may be replaced with frozen strawberries, raspberries, half a papaya or mango, or a few chunks of pineapple.

## Fruit Juice Smoothie

*2 cups apple juice*
*1 ripe banana*
*½ cup fresh or frozen strawberries or blueberries*
*½ cup pineapple juice*

Combine ingredients in a blender. Serve chilled.

## Energy Drink

*Dry mix*
*1 cup peeled almonds*
*1 cup sesame seeds*
*2 tablespoons protein powder (protein sources are from soy isolate [from soybeans], whey or casein [milk protein], and/or albumin [egg white])*

Combine ingredients in a blender, and blend until fine. This mix can be refrigerated for up to two weeks in a sealed jar. Blend with 8 fl. oz. of chilled fresh mix and drink as a meal enhancer or replacement. Use protein powder alone if other ingredients are not available.

*Fresh mix*
*1 ripe banana*
*1 cup fruit juice (apple, cranberry, or similar)*
*½ cup mineral water*
*honey to taste (optional)*

Combine ingredients with 1 tablespoon of the dry mix in a blender. Sip slowly.

You can add fresh berries to enhance canned products (Boost, Ensure, etc.).

## Immuno-Soup

This vegetable-based soup is high in immune-building nutrients. It is easily digested and makes a filling meal, despite being low in calories. It's also high in dietary fiber, which is supportive of colon health. A diet consisting of twenty-five to thirty grams of fiber each day improves the internal regulation of hormones. More than thirty-five grams may interfere with mineral metabolism and is not recommended.

*1 head celery*
*1 bunch parsley*
*½ pound green beans*
*4 zucchini*
*1 pound fresh spinach, beet greens, or chard*
*½ green bell pepper*
*½ red pepper*
*1 bunch scallions*
*1 large potato (Yukon gold are good)*
*3 medium carrots*
*½ head cauliflower or 1 head broccoli*
*1 turnip or rutabaga*
*1 parsnip*
*2 cloves minced fresh garlic*
*herbs to taste (thyme, rosemary, oregano, marjoram, etc.)*
*Any other vegetables are possible—experiment with seasonal and favorite varieties*

Wash, slice, chop, or grate all of the vegetables into even-sized pieces. Place root vegetables (carrots, potato, turnip, rutabaga, or parsnip) into a large pot. Half fill with water and bring to a boil. Cover and simmer for ten minutes. Add all the other ingredients and season to taste. Return to a boil and cook for another one to two minutes uncovered. Cover and simmer for another forty minutes. Adjust seasoning, and serve hot or cold.

*This soup improves with age. Cool rapidly, and keep refrigerated, or freeze serving-sized portions for a quick meal. Make sure you reheat thoroughly, and boil for at least two minutes when reheating. There are many anti-carcinogenic botanical factors or phytochemicals in vegetables, which help your immune system. This soup is a good way of getting your daily protection of plant-based nutrients. The soup contains less than three grams of fat (beneficial type).*

*Tamari, soy sauce, or Bragg's liquid aminos improve the flavoring. You can add more carbohydrate energy by adding brown rice, barley, noodles, canned beans, or corn. Serve with hot bread.*

Makes three to four bowls.

## Eating Tips During Cancer Treatment

Eating well is vital to give you that extra edge as you participate in your own recovery. Choose healthy foods to empower yourself for this important time in your life. Each time you choose a fruit, vegetable, or protein-rich food, you are giving your body what it needs to fight the cancer. Improved nutrition can also help you withstand the side effects of chemotherapy, radiation, and surgery. Some treatments may make eating difficult or distasteful.

Following are some specific suggestions to help you with some of the most common treatment-related problems. Even if some of these suggestions are in conflict with the basic high-fiber/low-saturated fat concepts with which you are familiar, maintaining a reasonably constant body weight is your overriding priority at this time. Fats or oils from sources that contain more of the beneficial fatty acids are useful to boost calories and still support your immunity. Examples include olives (and olive oil), avocados, nuts (almonds, walnuts, and Brazil nuts are particularly good, and nut butters are valuable ways of consuming them), and seeds (sunflower or pumpkin).

### For Chewing and Swallowing Difficulties:

- Eat foods prepared with moist heat (e.g., soups, stews, eggs, pastas, quiches, casseroles)
- Add gravy, sauces, butter, mayonnaise, or salad dressings to make food easier to swallow
- Avoid highly seasoned, spicy, tart, or acidic foods (no citrus fruits, tomatoes, chilies)

- Avoid alcohol and smoking
- Cold foods may be soothing if there are sores in the mouth. Use a straw
- Keep your caloric intake high by using meal replacement type drinks (e.g., Ensure)
- If you have trouble swallowing soups, try using a cup or glass instead of a spoon
- Carbonated drinks may be easier to swallow

### For Diarrhea:

- Avoid high-fiber foods that contain a great deal of roughage, e.g. whole wheat breads or cereals, raw fruits and vegetables (except bananas), cooked vegetables with seeds or skins, dried beans and nuts, and popcorn. Cucumber and lettuce may be difficult to digest
- Eat water-soluble, fiber-rich foods (e.g., applesauce or puree; psyllium, e.g. Metamucil)
- Don't drink with your meals, but drink plenty of water in between meals
- Eat frequent, small snack type meals, rather than three large ones
- Food and liquids should be warm or at room temperature, rather than very hot or ice cold
- For severe diarrhea, restrict your diet to clear, warm liquids such as broth, flat ginger ale, tea, or apple juice for one day. Check with your doctor if it persists more than one day

### For Nausea and/or Vomiting:

- Eat and drink slowly
- Eat small, frequent meals
- Avoid greasy, fatty, and fried foods
- Rest after meals
- For early morning or pre-meal nausea, try a cracker or dry toast
- Make up for lost calories when you feel more comfortable
- If cooking odors make you feel nauseated, try microwaving. Use a strong venting fan while you are cooking, or eat outside if the weather permits. Try frozen or chilled foods, as they give off less odor

*For Loss of Appetite*:

- If you aren't hungry at dinner time, make breakfast or lunch your main meal. Similarly, if you aren't hungry first thing in the morning, eat more later in the day
- Eat more frequently, but smaller amounts of food
- Keep snacks readily available in your purse or in the car
- Always make food look attractive with garnishes or place settings
- Experiment with tastes; you may find that things you didn't like before, you like now
- Cold or room-temperature foods may be more appealing
- A glass of wine or beer may increase your appetite (check with your doctor first, in case alcohol doesn't mix with a medication)
- Increase the caloric intake of the foods that you do eat with a small amount of "light" (less strongly flavored, not fewer calories) olive oil
- Try some of the commercially prepared food supplements such as Ensure, Boost, Sustacal®, or Polycose® powdered, unflavored starch, available from most good pharmacies or drug stores. Add fresh berries or juice for variety and additional botanical factors

## The Connection between Dietary Fat and Cancer

Recent studies indicate that many of the hormone-related cancers (breast, colorectal, and prostate) are linked to a high intake of animal protein and fat. It's prudent for those diagnosed with one of these types of cancer to cut back on dietary fat to about 20 percent of your calories from fat (about forty grams or about four tablespoons) with only 5 percent coming from animal sources (butter, milk, yogurt, meat, etc.) and 10 percent or more from fish or the plant kingdom (vegetables, nuts, seeds, and fruits such as avocados and olives).

Remember, too little fat is also harmful, and if you go lower than 15 percent of your calories from fat (about one to two tablespoons of oil per day) then use a supplement of borage or flaxseed oil for essential fatty acids, which are needed for proper brain and nervous function, as well as a healthy skin texture. A panel of nutritionists and scientists at the National Institutes of Health recently recommended that the ratio of omega-6 to omega-3 fatty acids should be four or less. Usual dietary intakes in the United States are much higher at 10–20:1. We can improve the ratio by cutting down on omega-6 and adding omega-3. Supplements of fish oil can help, especially if you don't enjoy eating fish.

If you've been diagnosed with another type of cancer, or you just want to eat a healthy diet, you should eat about 25 percent of your calories from fat—predominantly from fish or plant sources.

Omega-3 fatty acids are found in oily fish and some nuts, seeds, and vegetables. We eat fewer of these essential fatty acids in a typical modern diet, and recent studies indicate that we would benefit with supplementation. Evening primrose, flaxseed, and borage are good sources of GLA (gamma linoleic acid), which is also important in regulating hormones and prostaglandins (short-acting local hormones).

## Digestive Enzymes Explained

Digestive enzymes are proteins that assist in the breakdown of food components such as proteins, carbohydrates, and fats. The smaller fragments are made digestible, or able to be absorbed into the body, from the intestinal tract. Here's how it works: *Proteases* break down proteins, *amylases* break down carbohydrates, and *lipases* break down fats.

Bromelain, papain, and other proteases have been found to be beneficial to the immune system. Studies indicate increased numbers of white cells and activity of white cells when supplements of 250 mg or more are taken daily. Many people find that supplements of enzymes assist during chemotherapy, possibly helping to induce programmed cell death, or apoptosis. Bromelain is found in fresh pineapple, and papain comes from fresh papaya. Because enzymes are proteins, they are easily denatured by heat, which means they no longer do their work effectively because their shape is altered.

Why do we need to take enzyme supplements? Life today is so stressful that most of us don't secrete sufficient digestive enzymes. This results in intestinal discomfort and gas. Supplemental digestive enzymes can be helpful in reducing these symptoms, making you more comfortable during your cancer treatment.

## Exercise and Physical Activity

Exercise is the performance of physical activity that requires you to use energy. It's important to exercise as much as your condition allows, in order to keep your muscles functioning as well as possible. Exercise helps prevent problems that are associated with immobility, such as stiff joints, breathing problems, constipation, skin sores, poor appetite, and mental changes.

It's not unusual to lose strength and become de-conditioned as a result of cancer treatments, regardless of your previous level of fitness. Fatigue, pain, and the emotional adjustments that may accompany major changes in your body—such as being too weak to perform activities of daily living without assistance—may also take a toll. Many people have found that participating in some form of exercise helps them gradually to increase their endurance and ability to function more independently, which can have emotional benefits, as well.

Some things that may be helpful are to practice as much self-care daily as is comfortable, to take a walk every day, and to incorporate active or passive range-of-motion exercises as instructed by your nurse, doctor, or physical therapist. It's not in your best interest to stay in bed with little movement or to let others do for you what you can manage yourself.

Of course, you should contact your physician if you become progressively weaker, if pain increases, or if you have headaches, blurred vision, numbness, or tingling.

Some people may benefit from physical rehabilitation services that are designed to help you function as normally as possible. These services are carried out by physical and occupational therapists and rehabilitation counselors under the direction of a physician either in the hospital, an outpatient setting, or your own home. Physical therapy can help you to regain strength following major surgery; occupational therapy can help increase the strength and coordination of your body or to reevaluate your ability to return to your daily activities; and rehabilitation counseling can help you deal with the emotional impact of your disability.

In addition to physical benefits, participation in low-impact activities, such as yoga and T'ai chi, can help to focus the mind, alleviate tension and anxiety, reduce stress, and provide you with a renewed sense of wholeness and well-being.

In doing physical exercise, remember not to confuse "active" with "overactive." You need rest and relaxation during and after cancer treatments. Exhaustion can weaken physical and emotional defenses, and fatigue can make you feel depressed and discouraged.

## Taking the Best Care of Yourself

Because cancer treatment and fighting the disease can take all of your energy and then some, maintaining your health and wellness throughout treatment and recovery is essential. Attention to both can not only make you feel better, but also potentially ward off recurrence. It's absolutely critical that you monitor your diet, get lots of rest, and exercise as often as you can to keep your body and soul at their optimum cancer-fighting best.

**Patient Action Plan**
- Listen to your body's needs for rest and sleep
- You will benefit from being in natural surroundings and by keeping company with those who don't drain you of energy
- Because each person's nutritional needs are very individual, you should see a nutritionist or dietitian at this time to assist you in making healthy food choices
- Make a weekly food and exercise diary, and place it on the refrigerator. This way, you can monitor your changes in a way that's valuable for you, your family, and your health practitioners
- Remember to take extra care with personal hygiene at this time

## Chapter 16

# Facing the Uncertain Road Ahead
## Survivorship Blessings and Challenges

*I took more time for me and found that I was more important
to take care of at this time. It became easier to express feelings
toward family and friends. Every day is appreciated, rather than
being a drag. I enjoy my work but have time to do what makes
me happy. They say just thinking or planning something fun can
make your endorphins increase. I'm all for that!*

—DONNA PEDDICORD,
*participant, The Wellness Community - Valley/Ventura*

HE TERM "CANCER SURVIVOR" has different meanings for each person.
Being a survivor can refer to anyone diagnosed with cancer, regardless of the stage or course of the illness, and some people consider
themselves survivors from the time of diagnosis. Other people feel they
are survivors once treatments are over and they are either cured or in
remission.

Thanks to improvements in early diagnosis and treatment, some
forms of cancer have become more of a chronic illness for many people,
which means that you might have recurrent cycles of disease, treatment,
and then recovery. Relapse may occur in all types of cancer.

A lot of people have said that the fear of recurrence seems overwhelming, especially when treatment ends. The challenge is learning to live
in the moment and balancing the fear of recurrence with the desire to
enjoy health and wellness. It's during this period that people often find
support groups or individual counseling to be of the greatest value.

If you do experience a relapse, you may feel even more distress than
when you were first diagnosed. However, many people cope surpris-

ingly well with subsequent recurrences because they know what to expect, are more knowledgeable about treatment options and how to find support, and have learned to employ Patient Active strategies that help them retain control and hope. Staying Patient Active is your most important tool for long-term cancer survivorship.

> **Free *Cancer Survival Toolbox*® Available on iTunes**
> The award-winning *Cancer Survival Toolbox*, a patient tool from the National Coalition for Cancer Survivorship (NCCS), is now available on iTunes (www.itunes.com). The *Toolbox* is a free, self-learning audio program created by leading cancer organizations to help people develop important skills to better meet and understand the challenges of their illness.

## Dealing with the Reactions of Others

While you may be able to regain a sense of peace and balance despite the possibility of a recurrence, dealing with the feelings and opinions of others in your close circle may be another story.

Often, following the completion of cancer treatment, family and friends will encourage you to "get on with your life" and are seemingly unaware of the lasting impact that the cancer experience may have had on you. Many people with cancer often refer to the experience of living "A.C." (After Cancer) and never being able to return to "B.C." (Before Cancer). This may be a difficult concept for your friends and family members who want you to put the experience behind you.

It's important for you, as a survivor of cancer in whatever stage of treatment or recovery, to accept your feelings and find the places where it feels safe to express your feelings. It's also valuable to recognize that there are other cancer survivors who have fears and concerns that they may find it difficult to express to the well-meaning friends and family members who urge them to "put it behind" them.

But, as you are probably keenly aware, cancer isn't something anyone forgets. Anxieties remain as active treatment ends and "the waiting stage" progresses. A cold, a headache, or a cramp may be a cause for panic. As checkups approach, you, as well as family and friends, may swing between hope and anxiety. As time goes on and you wait for that magical five-year point, you may experience an increase in anxiety, rather than a feeling of stronger security.

There may also be long-term side effects from both the cancer and the treatment, which, depending on the type of cancer involved, can be as far-ranging as infertility to having a permanent colostomy. Being a survivor involves acknowledging and accepting these losses and changes. It also means understanding that there is a "new normal" for your life—and that this "new normal" is something faced not only by you, but also by almost all cancer survivors.

**LIVESTRONG™ Survivor*Care***
The Lance Armstrong Foundation's LIVE**STRONG** Survivor*Care* program offers counseling services; help with financial, employment, or insurance issues; and information about treatment options and new treatments in development. LIVE**STRONG** Survivor*Care* is for all cancer survivors, including those diagnosed, caregivers, family, and friends.

LIVE**STRONG** Survivor*Care* services include . . .
Cancer education:
- Information about cancer types and survivorship issues
- Treatment options
- How to find new treatments in development (clinical trials)

Help paying for treatment and other financial needs:
- How to pay for treatment if you are uninsured
- How to apply for Medicare and Medicaid
- Additional financial resources for insured patients:
  - How to manage insurance appeals and disability claims
  - How to make sure you have the coverage you need
  - Financial assistance for transportation, child care, and home care
  - Managing debt crisis issues

Practical tools and resources:
- How to manage your cancer experience
- Tips and tools for the caregiver
- How to find local resources and referrals
- Assistance with job retention and dealing with discrimination at work

Help with discussing your cancer:
- With your family
- With young children
- With your healthcare team

- With your employer
- With a support group
- With a professional

LIVE**STRONG** Survivor*Care* is a program of the Lance Armstrong Foundation in collaboration with Cancer*Care*, Patient Advocate Foundation, and EmergingMed.
For more information, visit www.livestrong.org, or call 1-866-235-7205.

*Source: Lance Armstrong Foundation*

## Coping with Changes

Even though friends and family members may suggest that you "forget about it," each person must seek individual ways of coping with whatever uncertainties and insecurities he or she has in being a cancer survivor. Here are a few suggestions for you from other cancer survivors:

- Get emotional, spiritual, and practical help if you need it, regardless of how long treatment has been over. Support groups, psychotherapy, educational workshops, rides to the hospital, spiritual counseling, etc., are all normal needs of people with cancer
- Find out about medications and mechanical aids to treat or reduce disability or discomfort, such as decreased mobility, sexual dysfunction, and other physical limitations
- Learn from others who have the same problems—join a support group, go to a class, and/or connect with someone who has had similar surgery or other treatments

*I'm so glad to be done...so grateful to be in remission. Cancer made me a better person....I'm forever changed, [but also] forever grateful for all of the awesome people who have blessed my life, both at The Wellness Community and beyond.*

—BECKY MORGAN,
*participant, The Wellness Community - Greater Lehigh Valley*

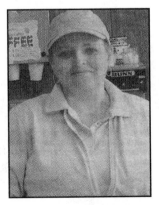

## Going Back to Work

While many people with cancer feel unable to continue with their normal employment during treatment, some people find that maintaining as much of their "normal" lifestyle as possible is extremely valuable. If you feel able to work, there's probably no reason why you shouldn't be able to do so.

The Americans with Disabilities Act (ADA) is a relatively new law that redefines disabilities to include cancer. Under the act, anyone who has had cancer is considered disabled. The goal of the ADA is to end job discrimination against people with disabilities, including discrimination regarding hiring, promotions, firing, pay, job training, and other aspects of work, including job benefits. A booklet from the American Cancer Society, "Americans with Disability Act: Legal Protection for Cancer Patients Against Employment Discrimination," provides a comprehensive overview of how a person with cancer might be protected by this law.

The Family and Medical Leave Act allows a patient or a family member caring for an ill person to take up to twelve weeks off from work without pay but with no loss of benefits.

Many cancer survivors need some physical rehabilitation before they are able to return to their old jobs or start new ones. Several different kinds of physical rehabilitation that might be helpful are:

- Physical therapy to gain strength and mobility
- Occupational therapy to increase strength and coordination of the body and to evaluate the ability to return to daily activities
- Rehabilitation counseling to help deal with the emotional impact of a disability

Employment rehabilitation may be needed if you decide to seek a different kind of work than you did before cancer. A person with cancer may be eligible for job retraining through the Vocational Rehabilitation Act of 1973, and there are employment agencies that can help with this process. The Office of Vocational Rehabilitation or a private employment agency can assist in finding out about these services.

## Seeking Legal Assistance

If you feel you've experienced discrimination in employment or insurance matters, you may decide to seek the advice of an attorney. It's advisable to contact a lawyer who specializes in employment or insurance law and has experience working with people who've had cancer.

Lawyer referral services are programs provided by a local or state bar association that are designed to help someone locate a private attorney to handle legal matters or problems. There may be a fee for the first consultation. The referral service may be able to help the person with cancer decide whether he or she needs to see a lawyer.

If you need a lawyer but cannot afford legal fees, a useful resource is the legal aid or legal services office in the county of residence. These offices handle some types of legal matters for people eligible under income guidelines established for their operation. The Patient Advocate Foundation (www.patientadvocate.org) may be helpful here if legal assistance is needed.

### A Prescription for Survivorship

No template exists for surviving cancer, so after treatment ends, many survivors go home without an understanding of what's next. Without a standard of care for monitoring survivors, they may not receive the necessary follow-up care needed to ensure the best quality of life and long-term survival. But some oncologists have stepped up and are pushing for a survivorship prescription for every person diagnosed with cancer. Following is an example of a survivorship prescription for a woman diagnosed with breast cancer.

**START: Primary care physician refers the patient to an oncologist to investigate lump felt in right breast**

**Step 1: Cancer Specialist: Diagnosis and Staging**
**Name:** Jane Doe

**Birthdate:** 4/13/1967

**Date of diagnosis:** 5/11/2006

**Diagnosis:** Stage 2A invasive ductal carcinoma; three of fifteen nodes positive; centrally located lesion

**Step 2: Treatment Summary**
**Surgery:** Lumpectomy and removal of three lymph nodes
**Chemotherapy:** Four cycles of Adriamycin/Cytoxan followed by Taxol

**Radiation:** Four weeks of radiation
**Hormone Therapy:** Five years of tamoxifen
**Complications/Side Effects:** Nausea and vomiting (grade 1);
hair loss; fatigue

**Step 3: Ongoing Care Plans**
*A. Long-Term and Late Effects Monitoring Needed:*
**Surgical:** Lymphedema (check arm for redness, swelling,
impaired range of motion)

**Chemotherapy:** Fatigue; minimal cognitive dysfunction; weight
gain; sexual dysfunction; increased risk of bone marrow damage
and/or heart dysfunction after anthracycline-based therapy

**Radiation:** Breast pain; muscle atrophy

*B. Surveillance for Recurrence:*
**Clinical:**
1. Monthly self-breast exam (report new lumps on breasts,
chest, and/or armpits)

2. History and physical breast exam every three to six months
after treatment for first three years, then every six to twelve
months for the next two years, then annually

3. Annual pelvic exam

**Imaging:**
Annual mammogram (women treated with breast-conserving
therapy should have their first post-treatment mammogram six
months after completion of radiation therapy, then annually)

**Surveillance for Secondary Cancers:**
Report bone tenderness; pain; cough; shortness of breath (data
not sufficient to recommend routine bone scans, blood counts,
or CT scans)

**Recommendations for Prevention:**
1. Genetic counseling
2. Exercise program/low-fat diet
3. Osteoporosis prevention therapy
4. Smoking cessation

**Psychosocial Issues That Need Addressing:**
1. Body image
2. Depression
3. Fear of recurrence

*C. Identify Physician Responsible for Monitoring Toxicity, Recurrence, and Other Issues:*
**Primary Care Physician:**
1. Address physical/emotional needs
2. Deliver chronic care needs that are feasible in the primary care setting
3. Refer for periodic evaluations and issues requiring specific expertise
4. Consult with specialists in areas of uncertainty

**Cancer Specialist:**
1. Provide guidance and specialized treatment as needed
2. Keep primary care physician informed of treatment plan
3. Option to return patient to primary care physician for implementation of plan and for care of other health needs

**Other Specialists:**
1. Genetic counselor
2. Dietitian
3. Physical therapist
4. Psychologist
5. Cardiologist

*Source:* CURE *magazine, Survivors Issue 2006. Used by permission.*

*At first, cancer was a bad word—but eventually, it becomes just another word. Take the capital 'C' off and you're not afraid of it.*

—ALFREDO DELAGARTA,
*participant, The Wellness Community - Greater Miami*

# When Cancer Comes Back

Let's face it: Cancer sometimes returns. When this happens, it's upsetting and challenging for you, your family, and your friends. The memories of doctor visits, treatments, surgery, or hospital stays can be overwhelming. If you have more problems with your cancer, it's natural to worry and feel down, knowing that you'll need more treatment, and that your future is once again uncertain.

You may feel like everything is spinning out of control again. Yet there are still things that you can do to regain control and manage the fears. There are often new medical treatments that are available, and your doctors will help you get the best care. It's also important to keep yourself involved with family, friends, and activities. This is one of the best ways to keep your mind in a positive place—by doing the things that you love.

"Taking one day at a time" has real value when you are faced with a difficult challenge. It's not just an old saying without meaning; it means keeping your mind focused on what you need to get done right now, today. Worrying about the future isn't the same as planning for your future, because it uses valuable physical and emotional energy; it prevents you from living your life now. You don't need to be a prisoner of your worries and concerns all the time. Keeping your mind busy doesn't mean you're in denial. It just means that you're allowing yourself to enjoy the rest of your life.

You are not your cancer. It's a huge part of your current struggle, but it isn't everything that you are. When you need to focus on medical issues, you can take care of business without getting overwhelmed by it all. Still, sometimes it's really hard to silence the worrying or negative voices you hear in your head.

Even if the cancer returns, and you have to deal with more illness and treatment, remember that doctors and scientists are working every day to come up with new treatment programs to help control cancer. If you need help getting through the tough times, your doctor or nurse can refer you to a therapist who knows how to help you regain your sense of balance and hope so that you can cope more effectively. You can also join a face-to-face support group or an online support group, such as those in The Virtual Wellness Community. In these groups, which are led by trained professionals, you'll connect with others who are going through the same things you are and learn ways to fight for recovery better.

## Uncertain Outcomes

The shock and dismay experienced by a person who is told that he or she has a diagnosis of cancer may be staggering, but for most people it's even more difficult to learn that their cancer has come back after some period of remission. Recurrent disease usually means more medical treatments, potential lifestyle changes, and, what may be even more frightening, concerns about the possibility of advanced disease and death. While cancer treatments after a recurrence may ultimately lead to a long-term remission or cure, for many people, a recurrence begins a phase of ongoing treatments where the outcome is less certain.

Sometimes, in spite of the best medical treatments and most conscientious self-care, cancer still recurs. The ways you and your family experience this event can be similar to how you dealt with it during the initial diagnosis. There's a need for decision-making with regard to new treatments, as the recurrence is dealt with medically, and often another period of acute care. The anxieties and fears of loss are often more intense than they were after the initial diagnosis because a recurrence seems more life-threatening, and it's hard to feel the same sense of hopefulness you may have had before.

It's important for you and your family to avoid looking for reasons for the recurrence. Despite popular literature to the contrary, there are no guarantees about preventing recurrences of cancer. No matter how much a person meditates, diets, prays, seeks treatments, etc., cancer may recur—and no one is to blame.

Survivors of most types of cancer may live with a series of recurrences or in chronic states of illness for many years. Having a constructive attitude and maintaining good communications can help you and those who care for you live as normally as you are all able. It can also be helpful for all involved to pursue individual interests, while developing and working toward mutual goals.

> **Creating an Ethical Will**
>
> Some people with cancer also make what is called an *ethical will*. It's not a legal paper. It's something you write yourself to share with your loved ones. Many ethical wills contain the person's thoughts on his or her values, memories, and hopes. They may also talk about the lessons learned in life or other things that are meaningful. They can say anything you want, in any way you want.
>
> *Source: "Coping with Advanced Cancer," National Cancer Institute, NIH Publication #05-0856*

## Advanced Cases

In situations where cancer has spread throughout the body—whether at the time of the initial diagnosis or after a recurrence—you, your friends, and your family must cope with the reality of advanced disease and the possibility of death.

Some terms that may be used by healthcare professionals to describe this situation are "terminal" or "end-stage disease." While this occurrence implies a finality that may be difficult to comprehend, it may be even more challenging to know that a terminal prognosis doesn't come with a timetable. Even when a doctor suggests that a person will live for a specific period of time, it's only an estimate. Some people who have advanced disease and are facing death have lived far longer than their healthcare team expected, and many are able to live their remaining days fully and with a renewed sense of purpose.

Like most people who feel emotionally distraught when they learn that their cancer can no longer be controlled, you may feel less able to cope with your day-to-day life and may even temporarily lose your will to live. However, feelings of hopelessness can give way to an inner strength you didn't know you had. You may start planning ahead for events that are weeks, months, or even a year in the future; looking forward to those events may even inspire you to live whatever time you have left to the fullest degree possible.

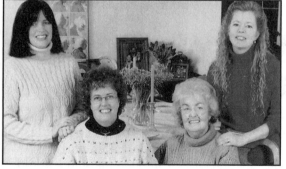

*Mary Varner, second from left*

*The way I see it is that, sooner or later, every one of us draws a death card. In my mind, cancer is not such a bad draw, because it gives you time to get your affairs in order and prepare your family…unlike, say, a massive heart attack or stroke.*

—MARY L. VARNER,
*participant, The Wellness Community - Delaware*

## Death and Dying—on Your Own Terms

It's normal for you and your loved ones to think about what you will face if the latest rounds of treatments aren't successful. Generally, a life-threatening illness prompts a re-examination of priorities to prepare the person with the illness and family members for the future and anticipate what they might need and want to achieve in the weeks, months, or even years ahead.

In thinking about death and dying, there are both emotional and practical issues to consider. Emotional issues related to preparing for death can include denial or anger that it is happening, depression and sadness that death is inevitable, and acceptance that death will occur. Having open, honest communication with your doctor and your family is a critical part of preparing emotionally and maintaining as much control as possible.

The practical issues pertain to getting your papers in order (*see Chapter 10*) to ensure that all of your wishes are carried out in the event of your death.

While few of us like to think about it, we all know that eventually death will come. Approaching death often brings about a change in how we view life, what we value, and how we relate to the people around us. There's no right or wrong way to face the end of life—as part of your own final expression, you'll do what's right for you. However, it may be valuable for you and your loved ones to consider questions about end-of-life care together and to proceed toward the end in a way with which each of you feels comfortable.

Honest and open communications are essential. Many people with advanced disease seek the help of professional counselors, spiritual advisors, and support groups to help them cope with the feelings they may have about their situations and to improve their communications with loved ones. It's important for everyone involved to have "safe places" where they can feel free to express their fears, frustrations, and concerns as the disease progresses and death becomes more imminent.

Finally, remember that even if you're okay with a potentially terminal outcome, not everyone can handle the grief and suffering of anticipated loss. Some friends may disappear, while other unexpected new sources of support may appear in your life. Stay as open as you can to all experiences—every interaction you have at this time of your life will be that much more meaningful in the end.

*I have made many wonderful friends, and I have lost many courageous friends. I feel a sense of purpose when I'm able to help other cancer patients navigate through the rough waters of a cancer diagnosis...my life has more meaning.*

—ALI DESIDERIO,
*participant,*
*The Wellness Community -*
*San Francisco East Bay*

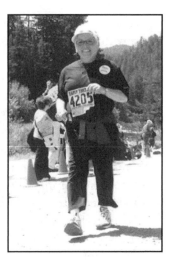

## The Hospice Option

Hospice care is one of the most useful resources that can provide care and comfort to the dying person and family members. Hospice care can be provided at home with specially trained nurses on call twenty-four hours a day. Hospice enables the person to stay at home and receive pain medication, oxygen therapy, skilled nursing care, and emotional support through educating and supporting the family in providing care.

The term "hospice" isn't new. Hundreds of years ago, a hospice was a place of refuge for travelers, often operated by a religious order, which provided comfort, kindness, and nourishment to people in need.

Most people, when asked, say that they don't want to die alone in a sterile, impersonal hospital room, hooked up by tubes to machines and cut off from the family and friends who are familiar to them. They also often say that they fear pain and suffering far more than they fear death. The modern concept of hospice was developed to address these concerns, fears, and anxieties of the person making the transition from life toward death.

You'll be eligible for hospice care when your cancer has become essentially unstoppable, and your death is generally expected within six months. But many physicians and families are uncomfortable addressing this likelihood, so they put off referrals to hospice programs until a person is near death. Unfortunately, at this stage, much less can be done to help the patient and family prepare and cope—which is why it's vitally important to discuss the option of hospice as early as possible as part of your end-of-life planning.

Hospice is committed to assisting the patient and his or her loved ones in many different ways that traditional healthcare may not, as follows:

- Hospice treats the person, not the disease
- Hospice offers palliative, rather than curative, treatment
- Hospice addresses the physical, emotional, social, and spiritual needs of the person with cancer and his or her significant others
- Hospice allows patients to spend their last days at home, alert and free of pain, among the people and things they love
- Hospice emphasizes quality rather than length of life
- Hospice offers help and support to the patient and family on a twenty-four-hours-a-day, seven-days-a-week basis
- Hospice helps family members and loved ones cope with the experience of the patient's dying

In addition, hospice provides continuing contact and support for family and friends for at least a year after the death of a loved one. Best of all, most insurance plans and Medicare cover the costs of hospice care.

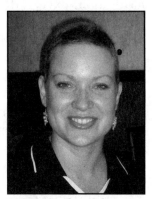

*Of course, I have limited control over my health. I decided to use this sad, hurtful time in my life to make lemonade out of lemons. It has been a great experience. I've met so many people, been able to give my testimony in hope for other women to be proactive and aware of their health. It's also made me realize what's important in life and what can wait.*

—Amy Matalka,
*participant, The Wellness Community -
Greater Cincinnati/Northern Kentucky*

## Finding New Meaning

Having advanced cancer can be challenging at first, but often gives way to a silver lining: You now have a chance to look back on your life and all you've been able to accomplish. Though there may be some regrets, most likely there are also many triumphs to celebrate—and many stories to pass on to others in your circle of family and friends.

Perhaps you're reflecting on just how much everyone in your life has meant to you. Or maybe you're honoring them in your own way for what they have become to you as you've traveled this difficult road together since the time of your diagnosis. Whatever's on your mind and in your heart at this moment, you've likely come to the realization that there's no better time than the present to create lasting memories for special people in your life.

In whatever form you choose to express yourself, creating living legacies can be therapeutic for you—and healing for those around you. The best part is, you needn't work on any of these projects alone, unless you choose to do so.

*A three-hour 'Healing Through Poetry' workshop led me to try writing poetry. Once convinced that I didn't need to know any of the 'rules of poetry,' I found I liked it [because] it enabled me to release some frustrations that I had buried. So far, I've written about twenty-five poems and continue to write.*

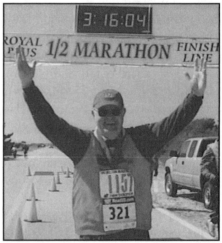

—DONALD H. WINSLOW,
*participant, The Wellness Community - Delmarva*

### Create a Living Legacy
Here are some examples of ways you can celebrate your life:
- Making a video of special memories
- Reviewing or arranging family photo albums
- Charting or writing down your family's history or family tree
- Keeping a daily journal of your feelings and experiences
- Making a scrapbook
- Writing notes or letters to loved ones and children
- Reading or writing poetry

- Creating artwork, knitting, or making jewelry
- Giving meaningful objects or mementos to loved ones
- Writing down or recording funny or meaningful stories from your past
- Planting a garden
- Making a tape or CD of favorite songs
- Gathering favorite recipes into a cookbook

*Source: "Coping with Advanced Cancer," National Cancer Institute, NIH Publication #05-0856*

## A Circle Journal of Love

For most people newly diagnosed with cancer, writing in a journal and keeping a photo album might be enough. But for David and Joan Frieder of Philadelphia, who had a blended family of several children and numerous grandchildren as far away as Vancouver, a journal that made the rounds to everyone seemed to make more sense. They started their "circle journal" in March 2001—almost one month to the day from when David was diagnosed with lung cancer.

The small, loose-leaf journal with a handmade paper cover in warm sage began with Joan's youngest daughter, Julie, who told David that she wanted him to dance at her wedding, though she hadn't even met her future husband yet. Two years later, he did exactly that.

The Frieders' circle journal became a labor of love for all of the members of Joan and David's family—even the youngest grandchildren, who wrote poems and pasted photos into the journal. The entries from others were just as poignant. Joan's daughter Sally once wrote: "You've always shown me how a father can really love his children and how a man can really love his wife. With your guidance, I could never settle for less. You've shown such bravery and character—both you and Mom with this new chapter in your lives. And, as with most things, you will be an example and mentor for us all to learn from, so that we will be better and stronger in the end. You both are my greatest friends. We are all here to help you fight. I love you both."

At first, the plan was for the children and grandchildren to fill in all of the pages, but it wasn't long before Joan and David began their entries, as well. "We couldn't help ourselves," Joan said. "We just had to see what everyone was writing in that journal."

More than any particular entry, David appreciated the overriding and powerful message that the circle journal conveyed: His cancer was, in fact, a family disease—and they were all together in the fight for his recovery, no matter where the journey might take them.

*Anything is possible, because I'm still here.*

—DAWN T. URSO,
*participant/volunteer,
The Wellness Community -
Philadelphia*

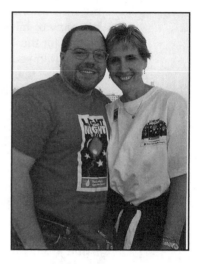

## Facing the Road Ahead

Harold Benjamin, our founder, advised early participants of The Wellness Community to continue to "make plans for the future." If you do so, then you're instantly recognizing that there's indeed still plenty of time left in your life. Wherever you may be in your treatment, thinking optimistically about the future is the key to survival. Your doctors and healthcare professionals are trained experts. By working closely with them on the best treatments available, as well as making plans for the future, however uncertain it may be, you're doing everything you can to get through your cancer experience with peace and dignity. In this way, you'll be the inspiration of all those who know and love you—and that's one very meaningful legacy.

**Patient Action Plan**
The small things that you do every day to maintain your normal routine will help prepare for the bigger challenges you may have to face in the near or distant future.
- **Keep moving ahead one step at a time.**
  Know that it might take a little longer to achieve everything you want
- **It's okay to feel overwhelmed by your concerns for the future.**

Perhaps you had your heart set on moving to another city or getting a new job, and now you're wondering if that will ever happen. Plenty of people have proven that your dreams don't have to come to an end because of cancer, but the "whens" and "hows" may need to be tweaked

- **It's okay to miss being with friends.**
  Plan for the time when you'll be with them again by seeing it in your mind, then breathe deeply to relax
- **Know that you're not alone and that there's indeed a future that will be rewarding.**
  Of course, you didn't ask for this challenge, but once you're in it, there's always something you can do to make a difference
- **Create some lasting ways to communicate your feelings** to your loved ones in the form of art, poetry, scrap-booking, or video
- **Prepare your will, living will, and advance directives ahead of time.**
  Many people with cancer find that this relieves them of some anxiety about how their wishes about dying will be honored
- **Communicate with your family and your doctor** about your needs, wishes, and expectations for end-of-life care
- **Discuss adequate pain control in advance** with both your doctor and your family
- **Seek out a counselor, spiritual advisor, or support group to explore feelings and concerns** about preparing for an uncertain future
- **Learn more about hospice care that's available in your area,** and talk with members of your healthcare team, friends, or other contacts to assess which one might provide the best care for your situation

# We Fight Cancer Together

*By Harriet Benjamin*

■ AM A THIRTY-FIVE-YEAR CANCER SURVIVOR. My husband, Harold Benjamin,
Ph.D., founded The Wellness Community in June 1982 as a result of
my experience with cancer. When I was first diagnosed, cancer was
whispered about or, worse yet, not even discussed. To many, it seemed
a death sentence.

Once I discovered that I had cancer, I really felt the divide. When I was
in the hospital, a wonderful woman from a cancer organization came to
visit me, and I told her I wanted to talk about my emotions...what I
was feeling. "Oh," she said. "We don't talk about that." It was because
of that experience that Harold and I realized there was a tremendous
need for a safe place to discuss what it means to have cancer and learn
whatever needed to be learned in order to fight for recovery. I came to
understand that isolation, hopelessness, and feeling out of control are
the most stressful aspects of cancer.

How very fortunate I was to have a caring, supportive community
surrounding me from that point on! They treated me like everyone else.
To them, I didn't have cancer—I was just one of them, part of an amaz-
ing group whose openness allowed me to laugh, cry, and express an
ever-changing range of emotions. From this solid foundation, I would
continue with my life—though never as a victim.

The world of cancer has changed tremendously since the early days
of The Wellness Community, but the needs of survivors have only
grown. Sadly, they will continue to grow. Fortunately for the survivors,
the story doesn't end there.

Today, as a result of The Wellness Community and many other important organizations, the patient advocacy movement has blossomed
into a force for great good in the world. No longer do people with cancer

or their families have to hide and feel isolated.

We are in this together—we fight cancer together. There are more avenues of support and more options than ever. This guide, which I hope you will keep with you and refer to often, provides an important road map for everyone touched by cancer. As my husband used to say, "We hope that everything turns out exactly as you want it to!"

At The Wellness Community, we'll continue to be there with you every step of the way.

# Improve the Quality of Life for Cancer Patients, Survivors, and Their Families

*We will support the development and dissemination of interventions to reduce the adverse effects of cancer diagnosis and treatment and improve health-related outcomes for cancer patients, survivors, and their families.*

THE NATIONAL CANCER INSTITUTE'S Vision to minimize the suffering and death due to cancer supports the interests of the more than ten million cancer survivors in the United States today. While the ultimate goal of eliminating cancer entirely continues to be our long-term commitment, the capacity to reduce dramatically the suffering caused by cancer is within our immediate grasp. This is in keeping with the Department of Health and Human Services Healthy People 2010 goal of five-year survival for 70 percent of those diagnosed with cancer. Advances in our ability to detect, treat, and support cancer patients have turned this disease into one that is chronic or readily managed for many and curable for increasing numbers.

We're learning more about the nature and scope of problems encountered by cancer survivors. Research is enabling us to predict who is at risk for adverse health outcomes better and to develop innovative interventions for treatment effects such as fatigue, memory difficulties, mucositis, nausea, and pain. Through clinical trials, investigators are trying to identify genes, proteins, or other biological markers associated with a patient's response to treatment. The ability to use genetic signatures to recognize tumors that are likely to recur after treatment could allow doctors to tailor treatment plans accordingly, sparing patients with good prognoses unnecessary therapy.

Partnering with others will assure appropriate follow-up care and increase adherence to optimal health behaviors among survivors. Understanding the impact of cancer on family members of patients and survivors—many of whom are themselves at increased risk for cancer due to shared cancer-causing genes, lifestyles, or toxic exposures—is also essential to achieving our Vision. As cancer care migrates to the outpatient setting, the economic, physical, and emotional burden on family members is increasing. Research must equip healthcare teams to prepare family caregivers better to manage patients at home while sustaining their own emotional and physical health.

STRATEGY 7.1—Expand research efforts to understand biologic, physical, psychological, and social mechanisms and their interactions that affect a cancer patient's response to disease, treatment, and recovery.

While research documenting the impact of cancer on patient and survivor health-related outcomes continues to grow, much remains to be learned about who may be at risk for specific disease- or treatment-related sequelae, what factors moderate or mediate risk, and the interaction of these on patient health. Increased understanding of how cancer patients respond to disease, treatment, and recovery will enable the development of interventions to improve quality of life during and after cancer treatment. NCI will:

- Strengthen behavioral and epidemiologic studies of cancer and its treatment among patients and survivors, examining both negative and positive physiologic and psychosocial effects and their correlates
- Support research on the biologic and physiologic mechanisms involved in adverse chronic and late effects of both current and new cancer treatments. Using molecular epidemiological research, we will seek to identify the genetic and/or phenotypic markers of susceptibility to treatment-related adverse effects and gene-environment interactions
- Promote the incorporation of quality-of-life endpoints within NCI-supported clinical trials and enhance the capacity for long-term follow-up of survivor cohorts
- Collaborate with others to synthesize the research on the role of

sociocultural, behavioral, emotional, and spiritual factors in survivor and family outcomes, and survivors' adoption of appropriate surveillance and health maintenance behaviors post-treatment

> **A World Forever Changed**
> As people emerge from the physical and emotional intensities of cancer treatment, they often find themselves in a world that is intimately familiar, yet forever changed. Typically, few signposts exist to guide these highly personal journeys. Survivorship research crosscuts the entire research portfolio to help chart and remediate that journey. We strive to adapt treatment to avoid chronic and late effects, ensure appropriate follow-up and post-treatment screening, prevent recurrence, and enable a high quality of life for cancer survivors and their families, friends, and caregivers.

**STRATEGY 7.2—Expand the development and use of tools to assess the health-related quality of life of cancer survivors and their family members across the trajectory of care.**

Improving patient outcomes will require tools to measure and describe patients' experience of illness, treatment, and recovery.

NCI will:

- Support the identification, development, and testing of instruments to assess the health-related quality of life of patients and survivors from diagnosis through the end of life
- Promote the routine use of standardized instruments at systematic time points across the trajectory of care, including the adoption of newly established criteria for monitoring harmful late effects of cancer treatment
- Collaborate with other NIH Institutes to support the development of measures and create data banks for evaluating comorbidities to better describe the effects of a cancer diagnosis on long-term health
- Support the development of measures to assess the impact of a patient's cancer on the health-related quality of life of family members and caregivers

STRATEGY 7.3—Accelerate intervention research designed to reduce cancer-related acute, chronic, or late morbidity and mortality.

As we learn more about the types and causes of adverse health-related outcomes among cancer patients and survivors, it will be critical that interventions to address them keep pace with our findings.

NCI will:

- Advance research on the most promising and cost-effective interventions to address cancer patient and survivor needs for improved quality of life—e.g., reducing cancer-related symptoms such as distress, pain, and nausea; minimizing post-treatment organ dysfunction; treating infertility; promoting healthy practices such as exercise, smoking cessation, and diet change; and addressing individual needs
- Support research to investigate the impact of well characterized and controlled interventions on appropriate intermediate biomarkers such as immune function, cortisol levels, and hormone levels
- Advance intervention development that promotes the health and well-being of family members and caregivers, as well as interventions that target patients and survivors in minority and medically underserved populations
- Foster development of screening tools that identify individuals or families at high risk for poor outcomes and support research to assess the impact of such screening on patterns and outcomes of care, including health-related quality of life
- Support the development of personalized treatments for individual patients based on their predispositions for adverse outcomes

STRATEGY 7.4—Ensure that relevant audiences receive new information, interventions, and best practices for addressing the health needs of survivors and their families.

As information becomes available about the nature of and ways to improve health-related quality of life outcomes for cancer patients, survivors, and their families, we must understand how to disseminate effectively this knowledge and evaluate its impact on care.

NCI will:

- Support the development and dissemination of curricula and standards for delivering effective psychosocial and supportive care for cancer patients and survivors to a broad spectrum of healthcare providers and cancer professionals
- Collaborate with other federal and health- or cancer-related professional and non-profit organizations and advocacy groups to promote the development and dissemination of educational materials across diverse media platforms—e.g., written, CD, audiotape, online, telephone—for family members and healthcare providers
- Assess health-related information needs and resources through patient, family member, and healthcare provider surveys and use this information to guide the development of educational tools and outreach efforts

## Actively Participate in Your Long-Term Well-Being

Because you know yourself best and will be the most knowledgeable about the history of your cancer treatment and care, it makes good sense for you to remain Patient Active in your long-term follow-up, as well—especially because some side effects don't show up for years.

As a long-term survivor, you need to be the primary person in control of your own health and personal well-being. But because some long-term health issues can be very complex, your support team, which can include your family, friends, doctors, and nurses, should also be actively involved every step of the way. (*See Chapter 16 for more on survivorship issues.*)

# References

## CHAPTER 5

*References*

*Chemotherapy and You: A Guide to Self-Help During Treatment.* National Cancer Institute, Publication No. 99–1136, September 1999.

Culkier, Daniel, M.D., Virginia S. McCullough and Frank Gingerelli. *Coping with Radiation Therapy: A Ray of Hope.* Lowell House, 1993.

Dodd, Marylin. *Managing the Side Effects of Chemotherapy and Radiation.* Prentice Hall Press, reprinted 2000.

G. Bonadonna, et al. *New England Journal of Medicine* 332 (1995): 901–906.

Gates R., et al. *Oncology Nursing Secrets.* Hanley & Belfus, Inc, 1998.

*Improving the Chemotherapy Experience.* Videotape and educational program, Amgen, Inc., 2000.

McKay, Judith and Nancee Hirano. *The Chemotherapy Survival Guide.* New Harbinger Publications, 1994.

*Radiation Therapy and You.* National Cancer Institute, Publication No. 95-2227, 1993.

## CHAPTER 7

*References*

*Alternative Medicine: Expanding Medical Horizons. A Report to the National Institutes of Health on Alternative Medical Systems and Practices in the United States.* Washington, D.C.: U.S. Government Printing Office; 1994. NIH publication 94–066.

Cassileth, B. *The Alternative Medicine Handbook.* New York, NY: W.W. Norton & Co., 1998.

Cassileth, B. and G. Deng, "Complementary and Alternative Therapies for Cancer," *The Oncologist* 9 (2004): 80–89.

## CHAPTER 9

*References*

1. Mock, V. (Chair), A. M. Barsevick, C. P. Escalante, P. Hinds, T. O'Connor, B. F. Piper, H. S. Rugo, et al. National Comprehensive

Cancer Network Clinical Practice Guidelines in Oncology, Cancer-Related Fatigue, Version 1.2006, 04-27-06.

2. T. J. Smith (Chair), J. Khatcheressian, G. H. Lyman, et al. "2006 Update of Recommendations for the Use of White Blood Cell Growth Factors: An Evidence-Based Clinical Practice Guideline," *Journal of Clinical Oncology*, May 15, 2006.

3. G. Bonadonna, A. Moliterni, M. Zambetti, et al. "Thirty Years' Follow Up of Randomized Studies of Adjuvant CMF in Operable Breast Cancer: Cohort Study." *BMJ,* 13 January 2005. < doi:10.1136/bmj.38314.622095.8F>.

4. B. Fortner, L. Schwartzberg, K. Tauer, et al. "Impact of Chemotherapy–induced Neutropenia on Quality of Life: A Prospective Pilot Investigation," *Support Care Cancer* 13 (2005): 522–528.

5. Rogers, G. M. (Chair), et al. National Comprehensive Cancer Network Clinical Practice Guidelines in Oncology, Cancer- and Treatment-Related Anemia, Version 2.2006, 04-19-06.

6. D. P. Friedman, "Perspectives on the Medical Use of Drugs of Abuse," *Journal of Pain and Symptom Management* 5(1 Supplement) (1990): S2–5. Available at http://www.cancer-pain.org/ treatments/addiction. html. Accessed on May 1, 2006.

7. Cancer Care, Inc., in cooperation with the Iowa Cancer Pain Relief Initiative and the Wisconsin Cancer Pain Initiative. Bill of Rights for People With Cancer Pain. Available at: http://www.cancercare.org/Pain/ PainList.cfm?c= 297. Accessed on October 1, 2003.

8. Ettinger, D. S., M. G. Kris, J. S. Stevens-Thorson, S. Raffine, J. McClure. National Comprehensive Cancer Network Nausea and Vomiting Treatment Guidelines for Patients. Version III. June 2005.

9. Holland, J. (Chair), et al. National Comprehensive Cancer Network Clinical Practice Guidelines in Oncology, Distress Management, Version 1.2005, 02-24-05.

10. M. Golant, "Managing Cancer Side Effects to Improve Quality of Life," *Cancer Nursing* 26 (2003): 37–46.

## Additional References

Benjamin, H. *The Wellness Community Guide to Fighting For Recovery from Cancer*. Putnam Press, 1994.

Holland, J., and S. Lewis. *The Human Side of Cancer: Living with Hope, Coping with Uncertainty*. Harper Collins, 2000.

## CHAPTER 11

*References*

1. Marcus, Amy Dockser. *Wall Street Journal,* April 6, 2004.
2. Marcus, Amy Dockser. *Wall Street Journal,* April 6, 2004.
3. Benjamin, Harold. *The Wellness Community Guide to Fighting for Recovery From Cancer.* Putnam Books, 1995.
4. Derogatis et al., 1983; Farber et al., 1984: Zabora et al., 1996.
5. J. Giese-Davis, C. Koopman, L. D. Butler, C. Classen, M. Cordova, P. Fobair, J. Benson, and D. Spiegel, "Change in Emotion Regulation Strategy for Women with Metastatic Breast Cancer Following Supportive-expressive Group Therapy," *Journal of Consulting and Clinical Psychology* 70(4) (2002): 916–925.
6. (A) Greenberg, L. "Emotion and Change Processes in Psychotherapy." In M. Lewis & J. M. Haviland (Eds.). *Handbook of Emotions.* New York: Guilford Press, 1993. 499–519.

   (B) M. A. Greenberg, C. B. Wortman, and Stone, A. A., "Emotional Expression and Physical Health: Revising Traumatic Memories or Fostering Self-Regulation?" *Journal of Personality and Social Psychology* 71 (1996): 588–602.

   (C) P. Salovey, A. J. Rothman, J. B. Detweiler, and W. T. Steward, "Emotional States and Physical Health," *American Psychologist* 55 (2000): 110–121.
7. J. Giese-Davis, C. Koopman, L. D. Butler, C. Classen, M. Cordova, P. Fobair, J. Benson, and D. Spiegel, "Change in Emotion Regulation Strategy for Women with Metastatic Breast Cancer Following Supportive-expressive Group Therapy," *Journal of Consulting and Clinical Psychology* 70(4) (2002): 916–925.
8. Marcus, Amy Dockser. *Wall Street Journal,* April 6, 2004.
9. Marcus, Amy Dockser. *Wall Street Journal,* April 6, 2004.
10. Groopman, Jerome. *The Anatomy of Hope: How People Prevail in the Face of Illness.* Random House, 2004.
11. Benjamin, *The Wellness Community Guide to Fighting for Recovery From Cancer.*

## CHAPTER 13

*References*

1. Weil, Andrew. *Eight Weeks to Optimum Health.* New York: Alfred A.Knopf, 1997; p. 250–51.
2. J. Giese-Davis, C. Koopman, L. D. Butler, C. Classen, M. Cordova, P. Fobair, J. Benson, and D. Spiegel, "Change in Emotion Regulation Strategy for Women with Metastatic Breast Cancer Following

Supportive-expressive Group Therapy," *Journal of Consulting and Clinical Psychology* 70(4) (2002): 916–925.

3. (A) Greenberg, L. "Emotion and Change Processes in Psychotherapy." In M. Lewis & J. M. Haviland (Eds.). *Handbook of Emotions*. New York: Guilford Press, 1993. 499–519.

   (B) M. A. Greenberg, C. B. Wortman, and Stone, A. A., "Emotional Expression and Physical Health: Revising Traumatic Memories or Fostering Self-Regulation?" *Journal of Personality and Social Psychology* 71 (1996): 588–602.

   (C) P. Salovey, A. J. Rothman, J. B. Detweiler, and W. T. Steward, "Emotional States and Physical Health," *American Psychologist* 55 (2000): 110–121.

4. J. Giese-Davis, C. Koopman, L. D. Butler, C. Classen, M. Cordova, P. Fobair, J. Benson, and D. Spiegel, "Change in Emotion Regulation Strategy for Women with Metastatic Breast Cancer Following Supportive-expressive Group Therapy," *Journal of Consulting and Clinical Psychology* 70(4) (2002): 916–925.

### Additional References

CancerCare Brief: *Strengthening the Spirit*. Cancer Care, Inc; 1998.

Hermann, F., et al. *Helping People Cope: A Guide For Families Facing Cancer*. Pennsylvania Department of Health, Cancer Control Program, 1988.

National Cancer Institute. *Taking Time: Support For People with Cancer and the People Who Care About Them*. National Institute of Health Publication No. 98–2059. (Revised September 1997).

## Chapter 14

*References*

F. I. Fawzy, N. W Fawzy, C. S Hyun, R. Elashoff, D. Guthrie, J. L. Fahey, and D. L. Morton, "Malignant Melanoma: Effects of an Early Structured Psychiatric Intervention, Coping, and Affective State on Recurrence and Survival 6 Years Later," *Archives of General Psychiatry* 50 (1993): 681–689.

D. Spiegel, J. R. Bloom, H. C. Kraemer, and E. Gottheil, "Effect of Psychosocial Treatment on Survival of Patients with Metastatic Breast Cancer," *Lancet* 2 (No. 8668) (1989): 888–891.

Spiegel, D., & Classen, C., *Group Therapy for Cancer Patients: A Research-Based Handbook of Psychosocial Care*, 2001, Basic Books, 303pp.

L. R. Derogatis, M. D. Abeloff, and N. Melisaratos, Psychological Coping Mechanisms and Survival Time in Metastatic Breast Cancer," *JAMA* 242 (1979): 1504–1508.

R. Gray, M. Fitch, C. Davis, and C. Phillips, "A Qualitative Study of Breast Cancer Self-help Groups," *Psychooncology* 6(4) (1997): 279–289.

B. McLean, "Social Support, Support Groups, and Breast Cancer: A Literature Review," *Canadian Journal of Community Mental Health* 14(2) (1995): 207–227.

R. W. Trijsburg, F. C. van Knippenberg, and S. E. Rijpma, "Effects of Psychological Treatment on Cancer Patients: A Critical Review, *Psychosomatic Med* 54(4) (1992): 489–517.

M. Glajchen and R. Magen," Evaluating Process, Outcome, and Satisfaction in Community-Based Cancer Support Research," *Social Work Groups*, 18(1) (1995): 27–40.

M. J. Cordova, J. Giese-Davis, M. Golant, C. Kronnenwetter, V. Chang, S. McFarlin, and D. Spiegel, "Mood Disturbance in Community Cancer Support Groups: The Role of Emotional Suppression and Fighting Spirit," *Journal of Psychosomatic Research* 55(5) (2003):461–467.

P. J. Goodwin, M. Leszcz, M. Ennis, J. Koopmans, L. Vincent, H. Guther, et al., "The Effect of Group Psychosocialsupport on Survival in Metastatic Breast Cancer," *New England Journal of Medicine* 345 (2001): 1719–1726.

B. Berglund, C. Bolund, U. Gustafsson, and P. Sjoden, "A Randomized Study of a Rehabilitation Program for Cancer Patients: The 'Starting Again' Group," *Psychooncology* 3 (1994): 109–120.

S. E. Taylor, R. R. Lichtman, J. V. Wood, A. Z. Bluming, G. M. Dosik, and R. L. Leibowitz," "Illnessrelatedand Treatment-related Factors in Psychological Adjustment to Breast Cancer," *Cancer* 55 (1985): 2506–2513.

Mahon SM, Cella DF, Donvoan MI, Psychosocial Adjustment to Recurrent Cancer. *Oncology Nursing Forum* 17(3 Supplement) (1990): 47–52.

V. Helgeson, S. Cohen, R. Schulz, and J. Yasko, "Education and Peer Discussion Group Interventions and Adjustment to Breast Cancer," *Archives of General Psychiatry* 56 (1999): 340–347.

C. Classen, L. D. Butler, C. Koopman, E. Miller, S. Dimiceli, J. Giese-Davis, R. Carlson, H.C. Kraemer, and D. Spiegel, "Supportive-Expressive Group Therapy and Distress in Patients with Metastatic Breast Cancer," *General Archives of Psychiatry* 58(5) (2001): 494–501.

M. Lieberman and M. Golant, "Comparisons between Internet and Face to Face Groups: The Expression of Fear and Anger in Breast Cancer Support Groups," *International Journal of Group Psychotherapy* (2004).

M. Lieberman, M. Golant, J. Giese-Davis, A. winzelberg, H. Benjamin, Humphreys, C. Kronenwetter, S. Russo, D. Spiegel, "Electronic Support Groups for Breast Carcinoma, A Clinical Trial of Effectiveness," *Cancer* 97 (2003): 920–925.

M. Lieberman, M. Golant, T. Altman, "Therapeutic Norms and Patient Benefit; Cancer Patients in Professionally Directed Support Groups," *Group Dynamic, Theory, Research and Practice*, 8(4) (2004): 265–276.

R. Gray, M. Fitch, C. Davis, C. Phillips, "A Qualitative Study of Breast Cancer Self-help Groups,"*Psychooncology* 6(4) (1997): 279–289.

B. McLean, "Social Support, Support Groups, and Breast Cancer: A Literature Review," *Canadian Journal of Community Mental Health* 14(2) (1995) 207–227.

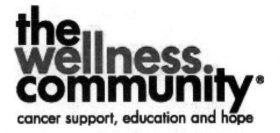

cancer support, education and hope

help@thewellnesscommunity.org
www.thewellnesscommunity.org

## National Offices
National Headquarters
919 18th Street NW
Suite 54
Washington, DC 20006
Toll free phone: 1.888.793.WELL
Ph: 202.659.9709
Fax: 202.659.9301

## Research & Development
11973 San Vicente Boulevard, #210
Los Angeles, CA 90049
Ph: 310.476.3727
Fax: 310.472.3161

## Quality Assurance & Facility Relations
445 East 71st Street
Indianapolis, IN 46220
Ph: 317.475.9321
Fax: 317.475.9338

## Online Initiatives
2111 Oakland Avenue
Covington, KY 41014
Ph: 859.581.3300
Fax: 614.413.3400

## Local Facilities

## ARIZONA
CENTRAL ARIZONA
360 E. Palm Lane
Phoenix, AZ 85004
Ph: 602.712.1006
Fax: 602.712.1009

## CALIFORNIA
FOOTHILLS
200 E. Del Mar
Suite 118
Pasadena, CA 91105

Ph: 626.796.1083
Fax: 626.796.0601

*Offsite Services of Foothills*
TWC at Providence
Burbank, CA

*Offsite Services of Foothills*
Las Palmas Community Center
San Fernando, CA

*Offsite Services of Foothills*
LAC+USC Women & Children's
   Hospital
Los Angeles, CA

*Offsite Services of Foothills*
Kaiser Permanente Medical Center
Baldwin Park, CA

*Offsite Services of Foothills*
Methodist Hospital
Arcadia, CA

*Offsite Services of Foothills*
Queen of Angels-Hollywood
   Presbyterian Medical Center
Los Angeles, CA

**ORANGE COUNTY**
540 North Golden Circle Drive
Suite 315
Santa Ana, CA 92705
Ph: 714.543.3200
Fax: 714.543.3327

**SAN FRANCISCO EAST BAY**
3276 McNutt Avenue
Walnut Creek, CA 94596
Ph: 925.933.0107
Fax: 925.933.0249

*Offsite Services of San Francisco/*
*   East Bay*
Bay Point Family Health Center
Bay Point, CA

*Offsite Services of San Francisco/*
*   East Bay*
Brookside Community Health
   Center
Richmond, CA

*Offsite Services of San Francisco/*
*   East Bay*
Concord Health Center
Concord, CA

*Offsite Services of San Francisco/*
*   East Bay*
Contra Costa Regional Medical
   Center
Martinez, CA

*Offsite Services of San Francisco/*
*   East Bay*
San Ramon Regional Medical
   Center
San Ramon, CA

*Offsite Services of San Francisco/*
*   East Bay*
Sutter Delta Medical Center
Antioch, CA

*Offsite Services of San Francisco/*
*   East Bay*
Sutter Solano Medical Center
Vallejo, CA

*Offsite Services of San Francisco/*
*   East Bay*
ValleyCare Health System
Pleasanton, CA

**SOUTH BAY CITIES**
109 W. Torrance Boulevard
Suite 100
Redondo Beach, CA 90277
Ph: 310.376.3550
Fax: 310.372.2094

*Offsite Services of South Bay Cities*
Long Beach Memorial Medical
    Center (LBMMC)
Long Beach, CA

*Offsite Services of South Bay Cities*
Torrance Memorial Medical Center
    (Lymphedema Support)
Torrance, CA

*Offsite Services of South Bay Cities*
Grupos al Harbor UCLA Medical
    Center
Primary Care Diagnostic Center
Torrance, CA

*Offsite Services of South Bay Cities*
Grupos al Harbor UCLA Medical
    Center
Torrance, CA

*Offsite Services of South Bay Cities*
Carson Community Center
Carson, CA

**VALLEY/VENTURA**
530 Hampshire Road
Westlake Village, CA 91361
Ph: 805.379.4777
Fax: 805.371.6231

*Satellite of Valley/Ventura*
Central Coast
San Luis Obispo, CA

*Satellite of Valley/Ventura*
Camarillo Healthcare District
Camarillo, CA

*Satellite of Valley/Ventura*
Cancer Center of Ventura City
Oxnard, CA

*Satellite of Valley/Ventura*
(Spanish Speaking)
Santa Rosa Catholic Church
San Fernando, CA

*Offsite Services of Valley/Ventura*
Centro Medico del Cordado de
    Ventura
Clinica de Oncologia/Hematologia
Cuarto Piso
Ventura, CA

*Offsite Services of Valley/Ventura*
(Spanish Speaking)
UCLA Medical Center
Sylmar, CA

*Offsite Services of Valley/Ventura*
(Spanish Speaking)
Our Lady of the Valley Catholic
    Church
Canago Park, CA

**WEST LOS ANGELES**
2716 Ocean Park Boulevard
Suite 1040
Santa Monica, CA 90405
Ph: 310.314.2555
Fax: 310.314.7586

*Offsite Services of West Los Angeles*
Cedars-Sinai Medical Center
Los Angeles, CA

*Offsite Services of West Los Angeles*
California Hospital
Los Angeles, CA

*Offsite Services of West Los Angeles*
LA County/USC Women's
    & Children's Hospital
Los Angeles, CA

*Offsite Services of West Los Angeles*
Hollywood Presbyterian Medical
    Center
Los Angeles, CA

*Offsite Services of West Los Angeles*
St. Vincent's Medical Center
Los Angeles, CA

*Offsite Services of West Los Angeles*
White Memorial Medical Center
Los Angeles, CA

*Offsite Services of West Los Angeles*
Kaiser Permanente Medical Center
West Los Angeles, CA

## DELAWARE

WILMINGTON
4810 Lancaster Pike
Wilmington, DE 19807
Ph: 302.995.2850
Fax: 302.995.0834

*Satellite of Delaware*
Dover, DE

*Satellite of Delaware*
Rehoboth Beach, DE

## FLORIDA

GREATER MIAMI
8609 South Dixie Highway
Miami, FL 33143
Ph: 305.668.5900
Fax: 305.665.0048

SOUTHWEST FLORIDA
3900 Clark Road
Building P-3
Sarasota, FL 34233
Ph: 941.921.5539
Fax: 941.921.5061

*Satellite of Southwest Florida*
Bradenton, FL

## GEORGIA

ATLANTA
5775 Peachtree Dunwoody Road
Suite C-225
Atlanta, GA 30342

Ph: 404.843.1880
Fax: 404.843.1780

*Offsite Services of Atlanta*
Northside Hospital—Cherokee
Canton, GA

*Offsite Services of Atlanta*
Northside Hospital—Forsyth
Cumming, GA

## INDIANA

CENTRAL INDIANA
8465 Keystone Crossing
Suite 145
Indianapolis, IN 46240
Ph: 317.257.1505
Fax: 317.254.4534

## MARYLAND

DELMARVA
1506 S. Salisbury Boulevard
Salisbury, MD 21801
Ph: 410.546.1200
Fax: 410.546.2542

*Offsite Services of Delmarva*
Regional Cancer Center
Easton, MD

*Offsite Services of Delmarva*
Ocean Pines Library
Berlin, MD

## MASSACHUSETTS

GREATER BOSTON
1039 Chestnut Street
Newton, MA 02464
Ph: 617.332.1919
Fax: 617.332.2727

*Offsite Services of Boston*
Dimock Community Health Center
Roxbury, MA

## MISSOURI

### GREATER ST. LOUIS
1058 Old Des Peres Road
St. Louis, MO 63131
Ph: 314.238.2000
Fax: 314.909.9900

## NEW JERSEY

### CENTRAL NEW JERSEY
3 Crossroads Drive
Bedminster, NJ 07921
Ph: 908.658.5400
Fax: 908.658.5404

## OHIO

### GREATER CINCINNATI/NO. KENTUCKY
4918 Cooper Road
Cincinnati, OH 45242
Ph: 513.791.4060
Fax: 513.791.8239

*Satellite of Greater Cincinnati*
Ft. Wright, KY

*Offsite Services of Greater Cincinnati*
The Barrett Cancer Center
Cincinnati, OH

*Offsite Services of Greater Cincinnati*
Christ Hospital Cancer Center
Cincinnati, OH

*Offsite Services of Greater Cincinnati*
The Allen Temple
Cincinnati, OH

*Offsite Services of Greater Cincinnati*
Mercy Hospital Western Hills
Cincinnati, OH

### COLUMBUS
5500 Franz Road
Suite 115
Columbus, OH 43017
Ph: 614.791.9510
Fax: 614.791.9610

## PENNSYLVANIA

### GREATER LEHIGH VALLEY
3400 Bath Pike
Bethlehem, PA 18017
Ph: 610.861.7555
Fax: 610.861.9177

### PHILADELPHIA
The Suzanne Morgan Center at
   Ridgeland
Chamounix Drive, West
   Fairmount Park
Philadelphia, PA 19131
Ph: 215.879.7733
Fax: 215.879.6575

*Satellite of Philadelphia*
The Ann McCouch Center
Lansdale, PA

*Community-Based Program of
   Philadelphia*
Tindley Temple United Methodist
   Church (TTUMC)
Philadelphia, PA

*Community-Based Program of
   Philadelphia*
Abbottsford Family Practice (AFP)
Philadelphia, PA

*Community-Based Program of
   Philadelphia*
Eastwick PAC (E-PAC)
Philadelphia, PA

*Community-Based Program of
  Philadelphia*
Haddington Multi-Services for
  Older Adults (HAD)
Philadelphia, PA

*Community-Based Program of
  Philadelphia*
Mercy Hospital of Philadelphia
  (MHP)
Philadelphia, PA

*Community-Based Program of
  Philadelphia*
Temple Hospital (TCC)
Philadelphia, PA

*Offsite Program of Philadelphia*
Grand View Hospital
Sellersville, PA

*Offsite Program of Philadelphia*
Hahnemann University Hospital
Philadelphia, PA

*Offsite Program of Philadelphia*
The Cancer Center at Paoli
  Hospital
Paoli, PA

## TENNESSEE

**EAST TENNESSEE**
702 Lindsay Place
Knoxville, Tennessee 37919
Ph: 865.546.4661
Fax: 865.522.0938

*Offsite Program of Knoxville*
Oak Ridge, TN

## INTERNATIONAL

**TEL AVIV**
The Wellness Community—
  Tel Aviv
(Beit Mati)

7 Revivim Street
Givatayim 53103 Israel
Ph: 972.3.731.5097
Fax: 972.3.571.9578

**TOKYO**
The Japan Wellness Community
Akasaka Berguo 805
3.11.14, Akasaka, Minato.Ku
Tokyo, Japan, 107.0052
Ph: 81.3.5545.1805
Fax: 81.3.5545.1806

## FACILITIES IN DEVELOPMENT

**CT: BRANFORD**
67 Turtle Bay Drive
Branford, CT 06405
Ph: 203.488.7549

**DC: GREATER WASHINGTON DC**
5430 Grosvenor Lane
Suite 100
Bethesda, MD 20814
Ph: 301.493.5002
Fax: 301.493.5004

**MI: SOUTHEAST MICHIGAN**
118 W. Jefferson
Ann Arbor, MI 48103
Ph: 734.572.0882 x 6
Fax: 734.663.9789

**NJ: NORTHERN JERSEY SHORE**
613 Hope Road
Eatontown, NJ 07721
Ph: 732.578.9200
Fax: 732.578.9201

**OH: DAYTON**
West Medical Plaza
1 Elizabeth Place, #110
Dayton, OH 45408-9901
Ph: 937.223.4117
Fax: 937.223.4118

Archie Bleyer, M.D.
  Medical Advisor
  Cancer Treatment Center, St.
    Charles Medical Center
  Bend, OR
Barry Bultz, Ph.D.
  Director of Psychosocial
    Oncology
  Tom Baker Cancer Center
  Calgary, Alberta, Canada
John R. Eckardt, M.D.
  Director of Clinical Research
  The Center for Cancer Care and
    Research
  St. Louis, MO
Luigi Grassi, M.D.
  Professor and Chair of Psychiatry
  Section of Psychiatry
  University of Ferrara
  Ferrara, Italy
Jimmie C. Holland, M.D.
  Wayne E. Chapman Chair in
    Psychiatric Oncology,
  Attending Psychiatrist
  Memorial Sloan-Kettering Cancer
    Center
  New York, NY
Paul Jacobsen, Ph.D.
  Director, Psychosocial &
    Palliative Care Program
  H. Lee Moffitt Cancer Center &
    Research Institute
  University of South Florida
  Tampa, FL

Matthew Loscalzo, MSW
  Associate Clinical Professor
    of Medicine
  Rebecca & John Moores Cancer
    Center, UCSD
  La Jolla, CA
John Marshall, M.D.
  Chief
  Division of Hematology/Oncology
  Vincent T. Lombardi Cancer
    Center
  Georgetown University Medical
    Center
  Washington, DC
Pearl Moore, RN, MN, FAAN
  (Retired)
  Oncology Nursing Society
  Pittsburgh, PA
Lidia Schapira, M.D.
  Assistant Professor of Medicine
  Harvard Medical School
  Massachusetts General Hospital
    Cancer Center
  Boston, MA
George Sledge, M.D.
  Professor of Medicine and
    Pathology
  Indiana University Cancer Center
  Indianapolis, IN
Kathryn M. Smolinski, MSW,
  LCSW-C, OSW-C
  Executive Director
  Association of Oncology Social
    Work
  Philadelphia, PA

David Spiegel, M.D.
  Jack, Lulu & Sam Willson
      Professor in the School of
      Medicine
  Department of Psychiatry and
      Behavioral Sciences
  Psychosocial Treatment
      Laboratory
  Stanford University School of
      Medicine
  Stanford, CA
Alan Valentine, M.D.
  **Deputy Chief of Psychiatry**
  University of Texas, M.D.

Anderson Cancer Center
Houston, TX
Jim Zabora, Sc.D.
  **Dean**
  School of Social Service
  The Catholic University of
      America
  Washington, DC

## Honorary Member
Fumiyoshi Takenaka, M.D.
  Founder and Executive Director
  The Japan Wellness Community
  Tokyo, Japan

**American Brain Tumor Association**
2720 River Road
Des Plaines, IL 60018
800.886.2282
www.abta.org
- Individual Counseling
- Peer Matching
- Patient Education
- Referrals
- Children's Services

**American Cancer Society**
1599 Clifton Road, NE
Atlanta, GA 30329
800.ACS.2345 (800.227.2345)
www.cancer.org
- Advocacy
- Support Groups
- Peer Matching
- Patient Education
- Referrals
- Medical Information
- Housing Assistance
- Transportation Assistance
- Financial Assistance
- Prevention/Detection
- Children's Services
- Survivorship
- Culturally Specific Resources

**American Hospice Foundation**
2120 L Street, NW
Suite 200
Washington, DC 20037
202.223.0204
www.americanhospice.org

- Advocacy
- Patient Education
- Referrals
- Hospice

**American Lung Association**
61 Broadway
6th Floor
New York, NY 10006
800.LUNG.USA (800.586.4872)
www.lungusa.org
- Advocacy
- Support Groups
- Patient Education
- Prevention/Detection
- Culturally Specific Resources

**American Pain Foundation**
201 North Charles Street
Suite 710
Baltimore, MD 21201
888.615.PAIN (888.615.7246)
www.painfoundation.org
- Advocacy
- Support Groups
- Patient Education
- Medical Information
- Culturally Specific Resources

**American Psychosocial Oncology Society**
2365 Hunters Way
Charlottesville, VA 22911
434.293.5350
www.apos-society.org
- Individual Counseling
- Referrals

**Angel Flight America**
4300 Westgrove Drive
Addison, TX 75001
877.858.7788
www.angelflightamerica.org
- Transportation Assistance

**Bladder Cancer Advocacy Network**
P.O. Box 341105
Bethesda, MD 20827
301.469.6865
www.bcan.org
- Advocacy
- Patient Education
- Financial Assistance

**Brain Tumor Society**
124 Watertown Street
Suite 3H
Watertown, MA 02472
800.770.TBTS (800.770.8287)
www.tbts.org
- Advocacy
- Support Groups
- Peer Matching
- Patient Education
- Referrals
- Medical Information

**BreastCancer.org**
111 Forrest Avenue
Suite 1R
Narberth, PA 19072
www.breastcancer.org
- Support Groups
- Patient Education
- Medical Information

**CancerCare**
275 7th Avenue
New York, NY 10001
800.813.HOPE (800.813.4673)
www.cancercare.org

- Advocacy
- Support Groups
- Individual Counseling
- Patient Education
- Referrals
- Insurance Information
- Financial Assistance
- Transportation Assistance
- Children's Services
- Survivorship
- Culturally Specific Resources

**Cancer Hope Network**
2 North Road
Suite A
Chester, NJ 17930
877.HOPENET (877.467.3638)
www.cancerhopenetwork.org
- Peer Matching
- Individual Counseling
- Referrals

**Cancer Information Services**
National Cancer Institute
Public Inquiries Office
6116 Executive Boulevard
Room 3036A
Bethesda, MD 20892
800.4.CANCER (800.422.6237)
http://cis.nci.nih.gov
- Patient Education
- Medical Information
- Prevention/Detection

**Cancer Liaison Program**
Office of Special Health Issues
Food and Drug Administration
5600 Fishers Lane HF-12
Room 9-49
Rockville, MD 20857
888.INFO.FDA (888.463.6332)
www.fda.gov/oashi/cancer/cancer.
html

- Individual Counseling
- Patient Education
- Referrals
- Financial Assistance

**Cancer Research and Prevention Foundation**
1600 Duke Street
Suite 500
Alexandria, VA 22314
800.227.2732
www.preventcancer.org
- Advocacy
- Patient Education
- Prevention/Detection
- Culturally Specific Resources

**Candlelighters Childhood Cancer Foundation**
3910 Warner Street
Kensington, MD 20895
800.366.2223
www.candlelighters.org
- Advocacy
- Support Groups
- Patient Education
- Referrals
- Medical Information

**Caring Connections**
National Hospice and Palliative Care Organization
1700 Diagonal Road
Suite 625
Alexandria, VA 22314
800.658.8898
www.partnershipforcaring.org
- Patient Education
- Referrals
- Hospice

**The Center for Mind-Body Medicine**
5225 Connecticut Avenue, NW
Suite 414
Washington, DC 20015
202.966.7338
www.cmbm.org
- Patient Education
- Referrals
- Medical Information

**Centers for Disease Control and Prevention Cancer Information**
US Department of Health & Human Services
1600 Clifton Road
Atlanta, GA 30333
800.311.3435
www.cdc.gov/cancer
- Patient Education
- Referrals

**Centers for Medicare and Medicaid Services**
US Department of Health & Human Services
7500 Security Boulevard
Baltimore, MD 21244
800.MEDICARE (800.633.4227)
www.cms.gov
- Insurance Information

**Children's Cause for Cancer Advocacy**
1010 Wayne Avenue
Suite 770
Silver Spring, MD 20910
301.562.2765
www.childrenscause.org
- Advocacy
- Patient Education
- Referrals
- Medical Information

**Clinical Studies Support Center**
National Cancer Institute
National Institutes of Health
  Clinical Center
10 Center Drive
Bethesda, MD 20892
888.NCI.1937 (888.624.1937)
http://ccr.cancer.gov/trials/cssc
- Referrals
- Medical Information

**ClinicalTrials.gov**
US National Institutes of Health
www.clinicaltrials.gov
- Referrals
- Medical Information

**Coalition of Cancer Cooperative Groups**
1818 Market Street
Suite 1100
Philadelphia, PA 19103
877.520.4457
www.cancertrialshelp.org
- Patient Education
- Referrals
- Medical Information

**Colon Cancer Alliance**
175 Ninth Avenue.
New York, NY 10011
877.422.2030 (helpline)
www.ccalliance.org
- Advocacy
- Peer Matching
- Patient Education
- Referrals

**Colorectal Cancer Coalition**
4301 Connecticut Avenue, NW
Suite 404
Washington, DC 20008
202.244.2906

www.c-three.org
- Advocacy
- Patient Education
- Referrals
- Medical Information

**Colorectal Cancer Network**
P.O. Box 182
Kensington, MD 20895
301.879.1500
www.colorectal-cancer.net
- Advocacy
- Support Groups
- Patient Education
- Peer Matching
- Referrals
- Screening

**Corporate Angel Network**
Westchester County Airport
One Loop Road
White Plains, NY 10604
866.328.1313
www.corpangelnetwork.org
- Transportation Assistance

**Emergingmed.com**
160 Madison Avenue
4th Floor
New York, NY 10016
877.601.8601
www.emergingmed.com
- Patient Education
- Referrals
- Medical Information

**ENACCT (Education Network to Advance Cancer Clinical Trials)**
1010 Wayne Avenue
Suite 710
Silver Spring, MD 20910
301.562.2774
www.enacct.org

**Family Caregiver Alliance**
180 Montgomery Street
Suite 1100
San Francisco, CA 94104
800.445.8106
www.caregiver.org
- Advocacy
- Support Groups
- Patient Education
- Referrals
- Culturally Specific Resources

**Gilda's Club Worldwide**
322 8th Avenue
Suite 1402
New York, NY 10001
888.GILDA.4.U (888.445.3248)
www.gildasclub.org
- Patient Education
- Referrals
- Individual Counseling
- Support Groups
- Culturally Specific Resources

**Group Loop**
The Wellness Community—
National
919 18th Street, NW
Suite 54
Washington, DC 20006
888.793.WELL (888.793.9355)
www.grouploop.org
- Support Groups
- Children's Services

**Inflammatory Breast Cancer Research Foundation**
321 High School Road, NE
Suite 149
Bainbridge Island, WA 98110
877.STOP.IBC (877.786.7422)
www.ibcresearch.org

- Advocacy
- Patient Education
- Referrals
- Culturally Specific Resources

**Intercultural Cancer Council**
6655 Travis
Suite 322
Houston, TX 77030
713.798.4617
www.iccnetwork.org
- Advocacy
- Patient Education

**International Myeloma Foundation**
12650 Riverside Drive
Suite 206
North Hollywood, CA 91607
800.452.CURE (800.452.2873)
www.myeloma.org
- Advocacy
- Support Groups
- Individual Counseling
- Peer Matching
- Patient Education
- Referrals
- Medical Information
- Culturally Specific Resources

**Joan's Legacy**
27 Union Square West
Suite 304
New York, NY 10003
212.627.5500
www.joanslegacy.org
- Patient Education
- Medical Information
- Financial Assistance

**Kidney Cancer Association**
1234 Sherman Avenue
Suite 203
Evanston, IL 60202
800.850.9132

www.kidneycancerassociation.org
- Advocacy
- Individual Counseling
- Patient Education
- Referrals
- Medical Information

**Kids Konnected**
27071 Cabot Road
Suite 102
Laguna Hills, CA 92653
949.582.5443
www.kidskonnected.org
- Support Groups
- Individual Counseling
- Peer Matching
- Patient Education
- Referrals
- Children's Services
- Culturally Specific Resources

**Lance Armstrong Foundation**
P.O. Box 161150
Austin, TX 78716
866.235.7205
www.livestrong.org
- Advocacy
- Patient Education
- Medical Information
- Survivorship
- Culturally Specific Resources

**Leukemia and Lymphoma Society**
1311 Mamaroneck Avenue
White Plains, NY 10605
800.955.4572
www.lls.org
- Advocacy
- Support Groups
- Individual Counseling
- Peer Matching
- Patient Education
- Referrals

- Medical Information
- Financial Assistance
- Transportation Assistance
- Culturally Specific Resources

**Living Beyond Breast Cancer**
10 E Athens Avenue
Suite 204
Ardmore, PA 19003
888.753.LBBC (888.753.5222)
www.lbbc.org
- Individual Counseling
- Peer Matching
- Patient Education
- Referrals
- Culturally Specific Resources

**Lung Cancer Alliance**
1747 Pennsylvania Avenue, NW
11th Floor
Washington, DC 20006
800.298.2436
www.lungcanceralliance.org
- Advocacy
- Support Groups
- Individual Counseling
- Peer Matching
- Patient Education
- Referrals
- Medical Information
- Culturally Specific Resources

**Lymphoma Research Foundation**
8800 Venice Boulevard
Suite 207
Los Angeles, CA 90034
800.500.9976
www.lymphoma.org
- Advocacy
- Individual Counseling
- Peer Matching
- Patient Education
- Referrals

- Medical Information
- Financial Assistance
- Transportation Assistance
- Culturally Specific Resources

**Melanoma Research Foundation**
24 Old Georgetown Road
Princeton, NJ 08540
800.MRF.1290 (800.673.1290)
www.melanoma.org
- Advocacy
- Patient Education
- Referrals
- Medical Information
- Prevention/Detection

**Men Against Breast Cancer**
P.O. Box 150
Adamstown, MD 21710
866.547.MABC (866.547.6222)
www.menagainstbreastcancer.org
- Peer Matching
- Patient Education
- Referrals
- Culturally Specific Resources

**Mesothelioma Information Resource Group**
205 Portland Street
Boston, MA 02114
888.802.6376
www.mirg.org
- Patient Education
- Referrals
- Medical Information

**MetaCancer Foundation, Inc.**
11 North Washington Street
Suite 600
Rockville, MD 20850
www.metacancer.org
- Support Groups
- Referrals

**Multiple Myeloma Research Foundation**
383 Main Avenue
5th Floor
Norwalk, CT 06851
203.229.0464
www.multiplemyeloma.org
- Advocacy
- Support Groups
- Patient Education
- Referrals
- Medical Information

**National Asian Women's Health Organization**
250 Montgomery Street
Suite 900
San Francisco, CA 94104
415.773.2838
www.nawho.org
- Advocacy
- Patient Education
- Referrals

**National Brain Tumor Foundation**
22 Battery Street
Suite 612
San Francisco, CA 94111
800.934.CURE (800.934.2873)
www.braintumor.org
- Advocacy
- Support Groups
- Peer Matching
- Patient Education
- Referrals
- Medical Information
- Culturally Specific Resources

**National Breast Cancer Coalition**
1101 17th Street, NW
Suite 1300
Washington, DC 20036
800.622.2838

www.natlbcc.org
- Advocacy
- Referrals
- Patient Education

**National Cancer Institute**
Public Inquiries Office
6116 Executive Boulevard
Room 3036A
Bethesda, MD 20892
800.4.CANCER (800.422.6237)
www.cancer.gov
- Patient Education
- Referrals
- Medical Information
- Prevention/Detection
- Culturally Specific Resources

**National Center for Complementary and Alternative Medicine**
National Institutes of Health
9000 Rockville Pike
Bethesda, MD 20892
888.644.6226
www.nccam.nih.gov
- Advocacy
- Patient Education
- Referrals
- Medical Information
- Culturally Specific Resources

**National Cervical Cancer Coalition**
7247 Hayvenhurst Avenue
Suite A-7
Van Nuys, CA 91406
800.685.5531
www.nccc-online.org
- Individual Counseling
- Peer Matching
- Patient Education
- Referrals
- Insurance Information
- Survivorship

**National Children's Cancer Society**
1015 Locust
Suite 600
St. Louis, MO 63101
314.241.1600
www.nationalchildrenscancersociety.org
- Advocacy
- Patient Education
- Referrals
- Insurance Information
- Financial Assistance
- Housing Assistance
- Transportation Assistance
- Children's Services

**The National Coalition for Cancer Survivorship**
1010 Wayne Avenue
Suite 770
Silver Spring, MD 20910
877.NCCS.YES (877.622.7937)
www.canceradvocacy.org
- Advocacy
- Patient Education
- Referrals
- Insurance Information
- Survivorship
- Culturally Specific Resources

**National Hospice and Palliative Care Organization**
1700 Diagonal Road
Suite 625
Alexandria, VA 22314
800.658.8898
www.nhpco.org
- Advocacy
- Individual Counseling
- Patient Education
- Referrals
- Medical Information
- Hospice

**National Lymphedema Network**
Latham Square
1611 Telegraph Avenue
Suite 1111
Oakland, CA 94612
800.541.3259
www.lymphnet.org
• Advocacy
• Support Groups
• Individual Counseling
• Peer Matching
• Patient Education
• Referrals

**National Marrow Donor Program**
3001 Broadway Street, NE
Suite 500
Minneapolis, MN 55413
800.MARROW.2 (800.627.7692)
www.marrow.org
• Advocacy
• Individual Counseling
• Patient Education
• Referrals
• Insurance Information
• Transplant Information
• Financial Assistance
• Housing Assistance
• Transportation Assistance
• Culturally Specific Resources

**National Ovarian Cancer Coalition**
500 NE Spanish River Boulevard
Suite 8
Boca Raton, FL 33431
888.OVARIAN (888.682.7426)
www.ovarian.org
• Advocacy
• Patient Education
• Referrals
• Culturally Specific Resources

**National Prostate Cancer Coalition**
1154 15th Street, NW
Washington, DC 20005
888.245.9455
www.fightprostatecancer.org
• Advocacy
• Patient Education
• Referrals
• Prevention/Detection

**Native American Cancer Research**
3022 South Nova Road
Pine, CO 80470
303.838.9359
www.natamcancer.org
• Patient Education
• Prevention/Detection
• Culturally Specific Resources

**NeedyMeds, Inc**
120 Western Avenue
Gloucester, MA 01930
215.625.9609
www.needymeds.com
• Referrals
• Insurance Information
• Financial Assistance

**North American Brain Tumor Foundation**
One Metro Center
700 12th Street, NW
Suite 900
Washington, DC 20005
202.508.4670
www.nabraintumor.org
• Advocacy

**Nueva Vida**
2000 P Street, NW
Suite 740
Washington, DC 20036
202.223.9100

www.nueva-vida.org
- Advocacy
- Support Groups
- Individual Counseling
- Peer Matching
- Patient Education
- Referrals
- Prevention/Detection
- Culturally Specific Resources

**Office of Cancer Survivorship**
National Cancer Institute
6116 Executive Boulevard
Suite 404
Bethesda, MD 20892
301.402.2964
http://survivorship.cancer.gov
- Patient Education

**Office of Minority Health Resource Center**
US Department of Health &
  Human Services
P.O. Box 37337
Washington, DC 20013
800.444.6472
www.omhrc.gov
- Patient Education
- Referrals
- Culturally Specific Resources

Oncolink
Abramson Cancer Center of the
  University of Pennsylvania
3400 Spruce Street
2 Donner
Philadelphia, PA 19104
www.oncolink.com
- Patient Education
- Referrals
- Medical Information
- Culturally Specific Resources

**Oral Cancer Foundation**
3419 Via Lido
Suite 205
Newport Beach, CA 92663
949.646.8000
www.oralcancerfoundation.org
- Patient Education
- Prevention/Detection

**Ovarian Cancer National Alliance**
910 17th Street, NW
Suite 1190
Washington, DC 20006
202.331.1332
www.ovariancancer.org
- Advocacy
- Patient Education Materials
- Referrals
- Medical Information

**Pancreatic Cancer Action Network**
2141 Rosecrans Avenue
Suite 7000
El Segundo, CA 90245
877.272.6226
www.pancan.org
- Advocacy
- Support Groups
- Individual Counseling
- Peer matching
- Patient Education
- Referrals

**Partnership for Prescription Assistance**
1100 15th Street, NW
Washington, DC 20005
888.4PPA.NOW (888.477.2669)
www.pparx.org
- Referrals
- Insurance Information
- Financial Assistance

**Patient Advocate Foundation**
700 Thimble Shoals Boulevard
Suite 200
Newport News, VA 23606
800.532.5274
www.patientadvocate.org
- Advocacy
- Patient Education
- Referrals
- Insurance Information
- Financial Assistance
- Medical Information
- Culturally Specific Resources

**The Patient/Partner Project**
P.O. Box 824
Twin Peaks, CA 92391
1.8.MORAL.SUPPORT
(866.725.7877)
www.thepatientpartnerproject.org
- Patient Education
- Peer Matching

**People Living with Cancer**
American Society of Clinical
Oncology
1900 Duke Street
Suite 200
Alexandria, VA 22314
703.519.2927
www.plwc.org
- Patient Education
- Referrals
- Medical Information
- Survivorship
- Culturally Specific Resources

**Planet Cancer**
314 East Highland Mall Boulevard
Suite 260-17
Austin, TX 78752
www.planetcancer.org

- Patient Education
- Peer Matching
- Children's Services

**Prostate Cancer Foundation**
1250 4th Street
Santa Monica, CA 90401
800.757.CURE (800.757.2873)
www.prostatecancerfoundation.
   org
- Advocacy
- Patient Education
- Referrals

**The Prostate Net**
835 Summit Avenue
Hackensack, NJ 07601
888.477.6763
www.prostatenet.org
- Advocacy
- Patient Education
- Prevention/Detection

**Rosalynn Carter Institute for Caregiving**
800 Wheatley Street
Americus, GA 31709
229.928.1234
www.rci.gsw.edu
- Advocacy
- Patient Education

**Sisters Network**
8787 Woodway Drive
Suite 4206
Houston, TX 77063
866.781.1808
www.sistersnetworkinc.org
- Advocacy
- Patient Education
- Prevention/Detection
- Culturally Specific Resources

**Skin Cancer Foundation**
149 Madison Avenue
Suite 901
New York, NY 10016
800.SKIN.490 (800.754.6490)
www.skincancer.org
- Advocacy
- Patient Education
- Referrals
- Medical Information
- Prevention/Detection
- Culturally Specific Resources

**Support for People with Oral and Head and Neck Cancer**
P.O. Box 53
Locust Valley, NY 11560
800.377.0928
www.spohnc.org
- Advocacy
- Support Groups
- Peer Matching
- Patient Education
- Referrals
- Medical Information

**Susan G. Komen Breast Cancer Foundation**
5005 LBJ Freeway
Suite 250
Dallas, TX 75244
800.IM.AWARE (800.462.9273)
www.komen.org
- Advocacy
- Individual Counseling
- Patient Education
- Referrals
- Prevention/Detection
- Culturally Specific Resources

**Thyroid Cancer Survivor's Association**
P.O. Box 1545
New York, NY 10159
877.588.7904
www.thyca.org
- Advocacy
- Individual Counseling
- Peer Matching
- Patient Education
- Referrals
- Culturally Specific Resources

**The Ulman Cancer Fund for Young Adults**
5575 Sterrett Place
Suite 340A
Columbia, MD 21044
888.393.FUND (888.393.3863)
www.ulmanfund.org
- Patient Advocacy
- Support Groups
- Patient Matching
- Patient Educational Materials
- Referrals
- Survivorship

**US TOO International Prostate Cancer Education & Support Network**
5003 Fairview Avenue
Downers Grove, IL 60515
800.80.US.TOO (800.808.7866)
www.ustoo.org
- Advocacy
- Support Groups
- Individual Counseling
- Patient Education
- Referrals
- Medical Information
- Prevention/Detection

- Culturally Specific Resources

**Vital Options International**
4419 Coldwater Canyon Avenue
Suite I
Studio City, CA 91604
800.477.7666
www.vitaloptions.org
  - Support Groups
  - Patient Education
  - Referrals

**The Wellness Community**
National Headquarters
919 18th Street, NW
Suite 54
Washington, DC 20006
888.793.WELL (888.793.9355)
www.thewellnesscommunity.org
  - Patient Education
  - Support Groups
  - Individual Counseling

- Referrals
- Medical Information
- Children's Services
- Survivorship
- Culturally Specific Resources

**Y-Me National Breast Cancer Organization**
212 West Van Buren
Suite 1000
Chicago, IL 60607
800.221.2141
www.y-me.org
  - Advocacy
  - Support Groups
  - Individual Counseling
  - Peer Matching
  - Patient Education
  - Referrals
  - Financial Assistance
  - Culturally Specific Resources

**Adoptive immunotherapy**: a form of treatment in development that uses a person's genes to instruct a human immune cell to find and destroy cancer cells.

**Aggressive cancer**: cancer that is fast growing.

**Alopecia**: hair loss. Alopecia is almost always temporary; hair grows back when therapy is finished.

**Anemia**: a shortage of red blood cells. This can cause weakness and fatigue.

**Angiogenesis**: the process of a cell developing new blood vessels.

**Anti-angiogenesis**: selectively stopping the process of angiogenesis by cutting off the support system of tumor cells.

**Antibody**: a substance made by B-lymphocytes that reacts with antigens (particularly proteins) on viruses, bacteria, and some cancer cells to mark them for removal.

**Anti-EGFR**: a new form of treatment that uses monoclonal antibodies that target members of the EGFR family in order to stop cell growth signals.

**Antigen**: proteins located on the surface of all cells. The immune system uses antigens to determine whether cells are a necessary part of the body or need to be destroyed.

**Apoptosis**: also called programmed cell death; a genetically determined process of cell self-destruction.

**B-lymphocyte**: a nearly colorless cell found in the blood, lymph, and lymphoid tissues that helps the immune system.

**Benign**: does not invade surrounding tissue or spread to other parts of the body; typically used to describe a tumor.

**Biologic agent**: a force or substance in the immune system that causes a change.

**Biologic therapy**: treatments that use or stimulate the immune system to fight infection and disease.

**Biopsy**: surgical removal of a small piece of tissue for evaluation under a microscope.

**Bone marrow**: the spongy material that is found inside our bones. It contains immature cells called stem cells that develop into three types of cells: red blood cells that deliver oxygen and take away the waste product carbon monoxide; white blood cells that protect from infection; and platelets that help the blood clot.

257

**Bowel perforation**: an emergency situation when the wall of the intestine or bowel develops a hole through its entire thickness.

**Cancer**: an abnormal cell that cannot be controlled by the body's natural defenses. Cancerous cells can grow and eventually form tumors.

**Cancer suppressor**: something that reduces or inhibits cancer growth.

**Cancer vaccine**: a treatment in development that helps the immune system to recognize cancer cells as harmful and therefore targets them for destruction.

**CD20 positive**: the presence of a specific antigen found on cell surfaces that helps in the growth and maturation of B-lymphocytes, which help the immune system.

**Chemoprevention**: using anticancer drugs to prevent certain types of cancer.

**Chemotherapy** ("chemo"): treatment with drugs to stop the growth of rapidly dividing cancer cells.

**Cytokine**: any of several regulatory proteins that are released by cells of the immune system and help in the generation of an immune response.

**Epidermal Growth Factor Receptors (EGFRs)**: see Human Epidermal Growth Factor Receptors.

**Familial adenomatous polyposis**: an often hereditary gene mutation that has been found to determine a person's predisposition to colon cancer.

**Fatigue**: a decreased capacity for mental and physical activity that is often accompanied by feelings of weariness, sleepiness, or irritability.

**First-line treatment**: generally the first standard therapy a patient receives upon initial diagnosis of cancer.

**Fluorescence in situ hybridization (FISH)**: a test to determine HER2 status; tags matching DNA—if more than one HER2 is tagged, there has been an increase.

**Gene therapies**: therapies that alter the genetic structure of tumor cells, making them more susceptible to either the immune system or chemotherapy drugs.

**Granulocyte-monocyte colony stimulating factor**: a certain cytokine that when increased, helps to boost a patient's white blood cell count.

**HER1 HER2 HER3 HER4**: a family of Human Epidermal Growth Factor Receptors that can indicate risk for excessive growth in certain cells.

**HER2 positive**: when there is an unusually strong growth signal from the HER2 receptor, causing the cell to grow and divide rapidly, creating an aggressive cancer.

**Heterodimerization**: the activation that occurs after two different receptors join.

**Heterodimerization inhibitors**: a group of agents that stops receptors from joining.

**Homodimerization:** the activation that occurs after two of the same receptors join.

**Human Epidermal Growth Factor Receptor (EGFR):** receptors found on the surface of both normal cells and cancer cells; members of this family are HER1, HER2, HER3, and HER4.

**Human Genome Project:** a project started in 1990 by the National Institutes of Health to identify genetic and environmental risk factors for all common diseases.

**Hybridoma technique:** laboratory methods that can produce a single antibody that recognizes a single antigen.

**Immune system:** one of the body's important defense mechanisms against infection.

**Immunohistochemistry (IHC):** a test done on a tissue sample of a tumor to determine EGFR status (usually for colon cancer).

**Immunotherapy:** see *biologic therapy*.

**Interferon alfa:** a protein released in the body in response to viral infections.

**Interleukin:** a group of natural, hormone-like substances produced by white blood cells in the body that play a central role in the regulation of the immune system.

**Intravenously:** administered into a vein.

**IV infusion:** when a drug is administered into a vein.

**Lymphocytes:** a type of white blood cell. Lymphocytes, carried along by the lymph fluid, are part of the immune system and fight infection.

**Metastatic:** a spreading of the cancer from the original tumor to different parts of the body.

**Monoclonal antibody:** a form of biologic therapy. Each monoclonal antibody acts specifically against a particular antigen.

**Mutation:** change.

**Neuropathy:** damage to the nervous system that can be caused by some chemotherapy drugs. Symptoms include weakness or tingling in the hands, feet, or both.

**Neutropenia:** an abnormally low level of neutrophils (the white blood cells responsible for fighting bacterial infections).

**Oncologist:** a doctor who specializes in treating cancer. Some oncologists further specialize in chemotherapy ("medical oncologists"), radiotherapy ("radiation oncologists"), or surgery ("surgical oncologists").

**Patient Active:** a concept at the core of The Wellness Community's program philosophy, which states that "People with cancer who participate in their fight for recovery along with their healthcare team, rather than acting as hopeless, helpless, passive victims of the illness, will improve the quality of their lives and may enhance the possibility of recovery."

**Pharmacogenomics**: the study of how an individual's genetic inheritance affects the body's response to drugs.

**Platelets**: a minute disk-like substance found in the blood of mammals that promotes blood clotting.

**Prognosis**: the likely outcome of a disease, including the chance of recovery.

**Proteomics**: the study of proteins found in cells, tissues, or organisms.

**Radioimmunotherapy**: a therapy that is prepared by attaching a radioactive isotope to a monoclonal antibody.

**Radioisotope**: see *radioimmunotherapy*

**Radiologist**: medical specialist who uses radioactive substances and X-rays in the treatment of disease.

**Receptor**: specific proteins on or inside a cell that can trigger the cell to do different things (divide, die, etc.).

**Regenerate**: to become formed or constructed again.

**Relapse**: the return of cancer after it has been treated and the patient has been in remission.

**Stem cells**: common cells found in the bone marrow (or peripherally in the blood) that are responsible for generating all the blood cells and platelets.

**Targeted therapies**: the newest category of cancer treatments that act in specialized ways to destroy or act against tumor cells and often avoid damaging normal cells.

**T-lymphocyte**: a type of white blood cell. Lymphocytes, carried along by the lymph fluid, are part of the immune system and fight infection.

**Tyrosine kinase**: an area within the human Epidermal Growth Factor Receptors (EGFRs) that is in charge of allowing cells to divide and multiply.

**Tyrosine kinase inhibitor**: a novel therapy in development that interferes with the cell signals found in the tyrosine kinase that tell the cell to divide and multiply.

**Vascular Endothelial Growth Factor (VEGF)**: a protein or growth factor involved in the process of angiogenesis.

**Vector**: a "vehicle" or carrier that transfers genes into cells during gene therapy.

## Personal Information

Medical Record Number: _____

Insurance Plan/Provider Number: _____

Type of Cancer: _____

Stage: _____

Date of Diagnosis: _____

Treatment Received to Date: _____

Your Personal Goals for Treatment: _____

_____

_____

_____

_____

| YOUR CANCER TREATMENT TEAM | | | | |
|---|---|---|---|---|
| Name | Specialty | Office Phone | Emergency Phone | E-mail |
|  |  |  |  |  |
|  |  |  |  |  |
|  |  |  |  |  |
|  |  |  |  |  |
|  |  |  |  |  |
|  |  |  |  |  |
|  |  |  |  |  |
|  |  |  |  |  |

## Quick Reference—Contact Numbers

Doctor_____

Phone_____E-mail_____

Doctor_____

Phone_____E-mail_____

Doctor_____

Phone_____E-mail_____

Nurse _____

Phone_____E-mail_____

Nurse _____

Phone_____E-mail_____

Nurse _____

Phone_____E-mail_____

Social Worker _____

Phone_____E-mail_____

Hospital_____

Phone_____E-mail_____

Ambulance_____

Phone_____E-mail_____

Pharmacy_____

Phone_____E-mail_____


Pharmacy_____

Phone_____E-mail_____


Insurance_____

Phone_____E-mail_____


Friend/Family Member_____

Phone_____E-mail_____


Friend/Family Member_____

Phone_____E-mail_____


Support Group_____

Phone_____E-mail_____

## Building Your Healthcare Team

Include your family or primary care physician, surgeon, medical oncologist, radiation oncologist, chemotherapy nurse, social worker, dietitian, physical therapist, etc. You may find it easier to tape business cards in your journal, so we have given you space to do that.

### *Your Hospital and Treatment Center Contacts*

Name_____

Address_____

_____

_____

Phone & Fax_____

E-mail_____

Specialty_____

Web site_____

Name_____

Address_____

_____

_____

Phone & Fax_____

E-mail_____

Specialty_____

Web site_____

## *Your Healthcare Providers*

Include your primary care physician, oncologists, nurses, and social workers.

```
┌─────────────────────────────────────────┐
│                                         │
│       Tape business card(s) here        │
│                                         │
│                                         │
│                                         │
│                                         │
│                                         │
└─────────────────────────────────────────┘
```

```
┌─────────────────────────────────────────┐
│                                         │
│       Tape business card(s) here        │
│                                         │
│                                         │
│                                         │
│                                         │
│                                         │
└─────────────────────────────────────────┘
```

Name_____

Address_____

_____

_____

Phone & Fax_____

E-mail_____

Specialty_____

Web site_____

Name_____

Address_____

_____

_____

Phone & Fax_____

E-mail_____

Specialty_____

Web site_____


Name_____

Address_____

_____

_____

Phone & Fax_____

E-mail_____

Specialty_____

Web site_____


Name_____

Address_____

_____

_____

Phone & Fax_____

E-mail_____

Specialty_____

Web site_____

Name_____

Address_____

_____

_____

Phone & Fax_____

E-mail_____

Specialty_____

Web site_____


Name_____

Address_____

_____

_____

Phone & Fax_____

E-mail_____

Specialty_____

Web site_____


Name_____

Address_____

_____

_____

Phone & Fax_____

E-mail_____

Specialty_____

Web site_____

*Your Medicare/Medicaid Plan*

Tape business card(s) here

Tape business card(s) here

Name_____

Address_____

_____

_____

Phone & Fax_____

E-mail_____

Specialty_____

Web site_____

Name_____

Address_____

_____

_____

Phone & Fax_____

E-mail_____

Specialty_____

Web site_____

Name_____

Address_____

_____

_____

Phone & Fax_____

E-mail_____

Specialty_____

Web site_____

Name_____

Address_____

_____

_____

Phone & Fax_____

E-mail_____

Specialty_____

Web site_____

Name_____

Address_____

_____

_____

Phone & Fax_____

E-mail_____

Specialty_____

Web site_____

Name_____

Address_____

_____

_____

Phone & Fax_____

E-mail_____

Specialty_____

Web site_____

## Outside Agencies and Organizations

Include visiting nurse/home health agencies, support organizations, and transportation services.

```
┌─────────────────────────────────────┐
│                                     │
│      Tape business card(s) here     │
│                                     │
│                                     │
│                                     │
│                                     │
└─────────────────────────────────────┘

┌─────────────────────────────────────┐
│      Tape business card(s) here     │
│                                     │
│                                     │
│                                     │
│                                     │
└─────────────────────────────────────┘
```

Name _The Wellness Community_____

Address_____

_____

_____

Phone & Fax_____

E-mail_____

Specialty_____

Web site _www.thewellnesscommunity.org_____

Name_____

Address_____

_____

_____

Phone & Fax_____

E-mail_____

Specialty_____

Web site_____

Name_____

Address_____

_____

_____

Phone & Fax_____

E-mail_____

Specialty_____

Web site_____

Name_____

Address_____

_____

_____

Phone & Fax_____

E-mail_____

Specialty_____

Web site_____

## *Other Important Contacts*

Include family and friends, neighbors, work associates, clergy, etc.

Name_____

Address_____

_____

_____

Phone & Fax_____

E-mail_____

Specialty_____

Web site_____

Name_____

Address_____

_____

_____

Phone & Fax_____

E-mail_____

Specialty_____

Web site_____

Name_____

Address_____

_____

_____

Phone & Fax_____

E-mail_____

Specialty_____

Web site_____

Name_____

Address_____

_____

_____

Phone & Fax_____

E-mail_____

Specialty_____

Web site_____


Name_____

Address_____

_____

_____

Phone & Fax_____

E-mail_____

Specialty_____

Web site_____


Name_____

Address_____

_____

_____

Phone & Fax_____

E-mail_____

Specialty_____

Web site_____

## Appointment Notes

Date: _____

Location: _____

With: _____

Questions I need to ask:

1.

2.

3.

4.

Action steps following this appointment:

1.

2.

3.

Questions I need to ask:

1.

2.

3.

4.

Action steps following this appointment:

1.

2.

3.

## Appointment Notes

Date: _____

Location: _____

With: _____


Questions I need to ask:

1.

2.

3.

4.

Action steps following this appointment:

1.

2.

3.


Questions I need to ask:

1.

2.

3.

4.

Action steps following this appointment:

1.

2.

3.

## Appointment Notes

Date: _____

Location: _____

With: _____


Questions I need to ask:

1.

2.

3.

4.

Action steps following this appointment:

1.

2.

3.


Questions I need to ask:

1.

2.

3.

4.

Action steps following this appointment:

1.

2.

3.

## Appointment Notes

Date: _____

Location: _____

With: _____

Questions I need to ask:

1.

2.

3.

4.

Action steps following this appointment:

1.

2.

3.

Questions I need to ask:

1.

2.

3.

4.

Action steps following this appointment:

1.

2.

3.

## Appointment Notes

Date: _____

Location: _____

With: _____


Questions I need to ask:

1.

2.

3.

4.

Action steps following this appointment:

1.

2.

3.


Questions I need to ask:

1.

2.

3.

4.

Action steps following this appointment:

1.

2.

3.

## Appointment Notes

Date: _____

Location: _____

With: _____

Questions I need to ask:

1.

2.

3.

4.

Action steps following this appointment:

1.

2.

3.

Questions I need to ask:

1.

2.

3.

4.

Action steps following this appointment:

1.

2.

3.

## Appointment Notes

Date: _____

Location: _____

With: _____

Questions I need to ask:

1.

2.

3.

4.

Action steps following this appointment:

1.

2.

3.

Questions I need to ask:

1.

2.

3.

4.

Action steps following this appointment:

1.

2.

3.

## Your Side Effect Tracking Log

A tool to help you track signs of infection and other treatment side effects during your cancer treatment.

### Date/Time/Treatment Cycle

Your doctor has planned several cycles of treatment for you, which will take place over a period of weeks to months. You can keep track of your schedule here.

### 1. Monitor Your Side Effects Every Day

Note any of the following symptoms. The symptoms that are <u>underlined</u> should be reported immediately. It is helpful to write your symptoms down to discuss them in detail with your doctor or nurse at your appointment:

- <u>Chills, sweating, fever</u>
- <u>Cough or sore throat</u>
- <u>Redness, pain, heat, or swelling around skin sores, catheters (port-a-cath, PICC line, etc.), or other wounds</u>
- Loss of appetite/ nausea
- Tingling sensation in fingers or toes
- Loose bowel movements/diarrhea
- <u>Shortness of breath or trouble breathing</u>
- Extreme fatigue or tiredness
- Dizziness
- Skin sores
- Numbness or tingling
- Loss of appetite or increase in appetite
- <u>Bruising or bleeding</u>
- Mouth sores, bleeding, or thick mucus
- Confusion, depression, or anxiety
- Nausea or vomiting
- Difficulty staying warm
- Pale skin
- Constipation
- Loss of or change in sex drive
- Pain (tell where)
- Rapid heartbeat

- Change in sleeping pattern
- Other

## 2. Medical Plan of Action

This should be based upon advice from your oncology team.

## 3. Personal Plan of Action

Include the steps you will take to resolve the problems you have discussed with your oncology team.

## 4. Other Solutions

Include any solutions not yet mentioned, including support groups, mind-body techniques, wellness techniques, or complementary medicine that you're interested in or currently use. (Please remember to tell your oncology team about any complementary or alternative medical and diet solutions that you use to ensure that they do not complicate your treatment plan.)

## 5. Record Your Blood Work Results

At office visits, your nurse may do a complete blood count, measuring the level of your neutrophils (infection-fighting white blood cells), hemoglobin, hematocrit, and platelets. These numbers tell your healthcare team whether you're at risk for side effects such as infection, fatigue, or bleeding. Write down the numbers your nurse gives you for the counts below:

Date:  Date the blood count was taken
ANC:  Absolute neutrophil count—measurement of infection-fighting neutrophils
Hgb:  Hemoglobin—measurement of the oxygen-carrying component of red blood cells
Plt:  Platelets—total number of cells that help stop bleeding
Other:  You may want to keep track of tumor markers or other tests that are specific to your cancer type and may be important to you

| Date/Time Treatment Cycle | 1. Side Effects | 2. Medical Plan of Action | 3. Personal Plan of Action | 4. Other |
|---|---|---|---|---|
| EXAMPLE Date: <u>July 10</u> Time: <u>4:15pm</u> Cycle: <u>1st Chemo.</u> | 1) 100.5°F fever 2) tired | 1) immediately call M.D. for fever 2) discuss fatigue at next appointment | 1) follow M.D. instructions 2) delegate tasks, find time for more rest | 1) try an on-line support group 2) try a low-impact exercise like yoga |
| Date: Time: Cycle: | | | | |
| Date: Time: Cycle: | | | | |
| Date: Time: Cycle: | | | | |
| Date: Time: Cycle: | | | | |
| Date: Time: Cycle: | | | | |
| Date: Time: Cycle: | | | | |

5.  Blood Work

Date: _____/___/_____

ANC: _____

Hgb: _____

Plt: _____

Other: _____

| Date/Time Treatment Cycle | 1. Side Effects | 2. Medical Plan of Action | 3. Personal Plan of Action | 4. Other |
|---|---|---|---|---|
| Date:<br>Time:<br>Cycle: | 1) 100.5°F fever<br>2) tired | 1) immediately call M.D. for fever<br>2) discuss fatigue at next appointment | 1) follow M.D. instructions<br>2) delegate tasks, find time for more rest | 1) try an on-line support group<br>2) try a low-impact exercise like yoga |
| Date:<br>Time:<br>Cycle: | | | | |
| Date:<br>Time:<br>Cycle: | | | | |
| Date:<br>Time:<br>Cycle: | | | | |
| Date:<br>Time:<br>Cycle: | | | | |
| Date:<br>Time:<br>Cycle: | | | | |
| Date:<br>Time:<br>Cycle: | | | | |

5. Blood Work

Date: _____/___/_____

ANC: _____

Hgb: _____

Plt: _____

Other: _____

| Date/Time Treatment Cycle | 1. Side Effects | 2. Medical Plan of Action | 3. Personal Plan of Action | 4. Other |
|---|---|---|---|---|
| Date:<br>Time:<br>Cycle: | 1) 100.5°F fever<br>2) tired | 1) immediately call M.D. for fever<br>2) discuss fatigue at next appointment | 1) follow M.D. instructions<br>2) delegate tasks, find time for more rest | 1) try an on-line support group<br>2) try a low-impact exercise like yoga |
| Date:<br>Time:<br>Cycle: | | | | |
| Date:<br>Time:<br>Cycle: | | | | |
| Date:<br>Time:<br>Cycle: | | | | |
| Date:<br>Time:<br>Cycle: | | | | |
| Date:<br>Time:<br>Cycle: | | | | |
| Date:<br>Time:<br>Cycle: | | | | |

5. Blood Work

Date: _____/___/_____

ANC: _____

Hgb: _____

Plt: _____

Other: _____

| Date/Time Treatment Cycle | 1. Side Effects | 2. Medical Plan of Action | 3. Personal Plan of Action | 4. Other |
|---|---|---|---|---|
| Date:<br>Time:<br>Cycle: | 1) 100.5°F fever<br>2) tired | 1) immedi-ately call M.D. for fever<br>2) discuss fa-tigue at next appointment | 1) follow M.D. instructions<br>2) delegate tasks, find time for more rest | 1) try an on-line support group<br>2) try a low-impact exercise like yoga |
| Date:<br>Time:<br>Cycle: | | | | |
| Date:<br>Time:<br>Cycle: | | | | |
| Date:<br>Time:<br>Cycle: | | | | |
| Date:<br>Time:<br>Cycle: | | | | |
| Date:<br>Time:<br>Cycle: | | | | |
| Date:<br>Time:<br>Cycle: | | | | |

5. Blood Work

Date: _____/___/_____

ANC: _____

Hgb: _____

Plt: _____

Other: _____

| Date/Time Treatment Cycle | 1. Side Effects | 2. Medical Plan of Action | 3. Personal Plan of Action | 4. Other |
|---|---|---|---|---|
| Date:<br>Time:<br>Cycle: | 1) 100.5°F fever<br>2) tired | 1) immediately call M.D. for fever<br>2) discuss fatigue at next appointment | 1) follow M.D. instructions<br>2) delegate tasks, find time for more rest | 1) try an online support group<br>2) try a low-impact exercise like yoga |
| Date:<br>Time:<br>Cycle: | | | | |
| Date:<br>Time:<br>Cycle: | | | | |
| Date:<br>Time:<br>Cycle: | | | | |
| Date:<br>Time:<br>Cycle: | | | | |
| Date:<br>Time:<br>Cycle: | | | | |
| Date:<br>Time:<br>Cycle: | | | | |

5. Blood Work

Date: _____/___/_____

ANC: _____

Hgb: _____

Plt: _____

Other: _____

| Date/Time Treatment Cycle | 1. Side Effects | 2. Medical Plan of Action | 3. Personal Plan of Action | 4. Other |
|---|---|---|---|---|
| Date:<br>Time:<br>Cycle: | 1) 100.5°F fever<br>2) tired | 1) immedi-ately call M.D. for fever<br>2) discuss fa-tigue at next appointment | 1) follow M.D. instructions<br>2) delegate tasks, find time for more rest | 1) try an on-line support group<br>2) try a low-impact exercise like yoga |
| Date:<br>Time:<br>Cycle: | | | | |
| Date:<br>Time:<br>Cycle: | | | | |
| Date:<br>Time:<br>Cycle: | | | | |
| Date:<br>Time:<br>Cycle: | | | | |
| Date:<br>Time:<br>Cycle: | | | | |
| Date:<br>Time:<br>Cycle: | | | | |

5. Blood Work

Date: _____/___/_____

ANC: _____

Hgb: _____

Plt: _____

Other: _____

## Personal Thoughts

Day/Date:_____

Time:_____


Personal Notes:

## Personal Thoughts

Day/Date:_____

Time:_____


Personal Notes:

## Personal Thoughts

Day/Date:_____

Time:_____


Personal Notes:

# Personal Thoughts

Day/Date:_____

Time:_____


Personal Notes:

## Personal Thoughts

Day/Date:_____

Time:_____


Personal Notes:

# Personal Thoughts

Day/Date:_____

Time:_____


Personal Notes:

# Index